Study Guide for

Clayton's Basic Pharmacology for Nurses

Eighteenth Edition

Michelle J. Willihnganz, MS, RN, CNE
RCTC Nursing Instructor
Rochester Community and Technical College
Rochester, Minnesota

ELSEVIER

ELSEVIER

3251 Riverport Lane
St. Louis, Missouri 63043

Study Guide for Clayton's Basic Pharmacology for Nurses, Eighteenth Edition   978-0-323-55473-2

Previous editions copyrighted 2017, 2013, 2010, 2007, 2004, 2001, 1997

Library of Congress Cataloging-in-Publication Data

Senior Content Strategist: Nancy O'Brien
Senior Content Development Manager: Ellen Wurm-Cutter
Senior Content Development Specialist: Rebecca Leenhouts
Publishing Services Manager: Catherine Jackson
Senior Production Editor: Claire Kramer
Design Direction: Renée Duenow
Publishing Services: Lisa Hernandez

Printed in the United States of America

Last digit is the print number: 9 8 7 6 5 4

Working together
to grow libraries in
developing countries

www.elsevier.com • www.bookaid.org

To the Student

This study guide was created to assist you in achieving the objectives of each chapter in *Clayton's Basic Pharmacology for Nurses, Eighteenth Edition,* and establishing a solid base of knowledge in nursing pharmacology. This study guide has been revised to emphasize the chapter objectives with NCLEX-style questions. Completing the questions for each chapter in this guide will help to reinforce the material studied in the textbook and learned in class. Such reinforcement also helps you to be successful on the NCLEX-PN.

STUDY HINTS FOR ALL STUDENTS

Ask Questions!

There are no stupid questions. If you do not know something or are not sure, you need to find out. Other people may be wondering the same thing but may be too shy to ask. The answer could mean life or death to your patient. That is certainly more important than feeling embarrassed about asking a question.

Chapter Objectives

At the beginning of each chapter in the textbook are objectives that you should have mastered when you finish studying that chapter. Write these objectives in your notebook, leaving a blank space after each. Fill in the answers as you find them while reading the chapter. Review to make sure your answers are correct and complete. Use these answers when you study for tests. This should also be done for separate course objectives that your instructor has listed in your class syllabus.

Key Terms

At the beginning of each chapter in the textbook are key terms that you will encounter as you read the chapter. The key terms are in color the first time they appear significantly in the chapter. Phonetic pronunciations are provided for terms that you might find difficult to pronounce. The goal is to help you if you have limited proficiency in English to develop a greater command of the pronunciation of scientific and nonscientific English terminology. It is hoped that a more general competency in the understanding and use of medical and scientific language may result.

Key Points

Use the Key Points at the end of each chapter in the textbook to help with review for exams.

Reading Hints

When reading each chapter in the textbook, look at the subject headings to learn what each section is about. Read first for the general meaning. Then reread parts you did not understand. It may help to read those parts aloud. Carefully read the information given in each table and study each figure and its caption.

Concepts

While studying, put difficult concepts into your own words to see if you understand them. Check this understanding with another student or the instructor. Write these in your notebook.

Class Notes

When taking lecture notes in class, leave a large margin on the left side of each notebook page and write only on right-hand pages, leaving all left-hand pages blank. Look over your lecture notes soon after each class, while your memory is fresh. Fill in missing words, complete sentences and ideas, and underline key phrases, definitions, and concepts. At the top of each page, write the topic of that page. In the left margin, write the key word for that part of your notes. On the opposite left-hand page, write a summary or outline that combines material from both the textbook and the lecture. These can be your study notes for review.

Study Groups

Form a study group with some other students so you can help one another. Practice speaking and reading aloud. Ask questions about material you are not sure about. Work together to find answers.

References for Improving Study Skills

Good study skills are essential for achieving your goals in nursing. Time management, efficient use of study time, and a consistent approach to studying are all beneficial. There are various study methods for reading a textbook and for taking class notes. Some methods that have proven helpful can be found in *Saunders Student Nurse Planner: A Guide to Success in Nursing School.* This book contains helpful information on test taking and preparing for clinical experiences. It includes an example of a "time map" for planning study time and a blank form that you can use to formulate a personal time map.

ADDITIONAL STUDY HINTS FOR ENGLISH AS SECOND-LANGUAGE (ESL) STUDENTS

Vocabulary

If you find a nontechnical word you do not know (e.g., *drowsy*), try to guess its meaning from the sentence (e.g., *With electrolyte imbalance, the patient may feel fatigued and drowsy*). If you are not sure of the meaning, or if it seems particularly important, look it up in the dictionary.

Vocabulary Notebook

Keep a small alphabetized notebook or address book in your pocket or purse. Write down new nontechnical words you read or hear along with their meanings and pronunciations. Write each word under its initial letter so you can find it easily, as in a dictionary. For words you do not know or for words that have a different meaning in nursing, write down how they are used and sound. Look up their meanings in a dictionary or ask your instructor or first-language buddy. Then write the different meanings or usages that you have found in your book, including the nursing meaning. Continue to add new words as you discover them. For example:

primary
- of most importance; main: *the primary problem or disease*
- the first one; elementary: *primary school*

secondary
- of less importance; resulting from another problem or disease: *a secondary symptom*
- the second one: *secondary school (in the United States, high school)*

First Language Buddy

ESL students should find a first-language buddy – another student who is a native speaker of English and who is willing to answer questions about word meanings, pronunciations, and culture. Maybe your buddy would like to learn about your language and culture also. This could help in his or her nursing experience as well.

Contents

Drug Definitions, Standards, and Information Sources

chapter **1**

Answer Key: Textbook page references are provided as a guide for answering these questions. A complete answer key is provided to your instructor.

MATCHING
Match the drug schedule on the right with the drug name on the left.

Drug

1. _____ diazepam (Valium)
2. _____ guaifenesin (Robitussin AC)
3. _____ heroin
4. _____ hydrocodone and Tylenol (Norco)
5. _____ methylphenidate (Ritalin)

Drug Schedule (U.S. Only)

a. Schedule I
b. Schedule II
c. Schedule III
d. Schedule IV
e. Schedule V

REVIEW QUESTIONS

Differentiate among the chemical, generic, and brand names of drugs.

6. Chemical names of drugs are used for which purpose? *(2)*
   1. To describe the exact chemical makeup of the drug.
   2. To provide a simpler way to identify the drug being manufactured.
   3. To market the drug to the public.
   4. To identify illegal drugs.
7. Generic names of drugs are used for which purpose? *(2)*
   1. To describe the exact chemical makeup of the drug.
   2. To provide a simpler way to identify the drug being manufactured.
   3. To market the drug to the public.
   4. To identify illegal drugs.
8. Brand names of drugs are used for which purpose? *(2)*
   1. To describe the exact chemical makeup of the drug.
   2. To provide a simpler way to identify the drug being manufactured.
   3. To market the drug to the public.
   4. To identify illegal drugs.

9. The drug Zyrtec is an example of what type of drug name? *(2)*
   1. The chemical name of the drug.
   2. The brand name of the drug.
   3. The generic name of the drug.
   4. The illegal name of the drug.

Identify the various methods used to classify drugs.

10. While studying drugs in school, the nursing student learns that the methods used to classify drugs includes the drug's: *(Select all that apply.) (2)*
    1. chemical action.
    2. effect on a body system.
    3. therapeutic use.
    4. clinical indication.
    5. route of administration.
11. Examples of drugs that are classified by their physiologic or chemical action include which classification(s)? *(Select all that apply.) (2)*
    1. Anticholinergics
    2. Antacids
    3. Antibiotics
    4. Beta-adrenergic blockers
    5. Antihypertensives
12. When drugs are classified according to body systems, their effect can involve which system? *(Select all that apply.) (2)*
    1. Cardiovascular system
    2. Respiratory system
    3. Nervous system
    4. Apothecary system
    5. Metric system

13. The patient asks a nurse what the difference is between biosimilars and generic biologic agents. The nurse responds with which appropriate statement? *(2)*
    1. "As I understand it, the biosimilars are exactly the same as the generic biologic agents, only cheaper."
    2. "The biosimilar agents are manufactured to replace the biologic agents because they are smaller and less complex drugs."
    3. "The biosimilars are close in structure and function to biologics but not identical."
    4. "The biosimilars are more expensive and have predictable reactions compared to biologics."

Identify sources of drug information available for healthcare providers.

14. Which resources are the most useful for nurses seeking information about prescription medications? *(Select all that apply.) (4)*
    1. Natural Medicines Comprehensive Database
    2. *Physician's Drug Reference*
    3. American Hospital Formulary Service, Drug Information
    4. Drug Interaction Facts
    5. Drug Facts and Comparisons

15. Which would be considered a reliable database for drug information that a nurse can consult? *(Select all that apply.) (3)*
    1. *Handbook of Nonprescription Drugs: An Interactive Approach to Self-Care*
    2. *United States Pharmacopeia (USP)/National Formulary (NF)*
    3. Lexi-Comp
    4. Electronic databases such as CINAHL
    5. ePocrates

16. A patient has been experiencing adverse effects from a hypertensive medication he was prescribed. The nurse realizes that this adverse effect will need to be reported through which program? *(8)*
    1. Watchman program
    2. MedWatch program
    3. PharmWatch program
    4. DrugWatch program

17. A nurse is preparing a scholarly publication on the responses to and adverse effects of heparin. The most efficient and effective means of gathering information for this publication is to use which source? *(3)*
    1. Package inserts from drugs
    2. A consumer health website
    3. Wikipedia
    4. CINAHL database

18. As a healthcare professional, it is important that the nurse determine the most accurate and up-to-date Internet information available for drugs that includes which sites? *(Select all that apply.) (3)*
    1. ePocrates
    2. DailyMed
    3. Yahoo
    4. Lexi-Comp
    5. Krames Online

Cite sources of credible drug information on the Internet.

19. A patient asked the nurse where to find information about the drug she was prescribed. The nurse responds with which appropriate statement? *(19)*
    1. "Ask your healthcare provider to discuss your case in detail. The Internet can be misleading."
    2. "The best source for drug information is just to Google it."
    3. "We will give you all of the information you will need about your medications; you do not have to look any further."
    4. "A variety of sources are available to you. We will provide information, you can ask your healthcare provider, and you can research information online."

20. The nurse understands that a credible source of drug information on the Internet includes which site? *(20)*
    1. Health on the Net Foundation
    2. Google
    3. Wikipedia
    4. Drugs, Inc.

21. The nurse explaining to a patient sources for drug information on the Internet discusses a searchable database developed in collaboration with federal agencies such as the FDA that allows users to get more information. This database is known as: *(3)*
    1. ePocrates.
    2. Wikipedia.
    3. DailyMed.
    4. DART.

Discuss the difference between prescription and nonprescription drugs.

22. The difference between prescription and nonprescription drugs is that prescription drugs: *(2)*
    1. are generally cheaper than nonprescription drugs.
    2. need to be obtained through a licensed healthcare provider.
    3. are identified using the brand name and nonprescription drugs use the generic name.
    4. do not have any serious side effects.

23. A patient asks the nurse what the difference is between prescription and nonprescription drugs. What is the best response by the nurse? *(2)*
    1. "The difference between the two classifications is really complicated and you just need to follow your healthcare provider's advice."
    2. "Any store that has medications on the shelves indicates that you can purchase them without a prescription."
    3. "The difference between these two types of drugs is that one is the brand name and the other is the generic name."
    4. "Nonprescription drugs do not need to be approved by the FDA and prescription drugs do."
24. Which healthcare providers are licensed to prescribe drugs? *(Select all that apply.) (2)*
    1. Pharmacists
    2. Nurses
    3. Physicians
    4. Dentists
    5. Physician assistant

Describe the process of developing and bringing new drugs to market.

25. Those patients who participate in "testing in humans" are part of which phase of new drug development? *(8)*
    1. Preclinical research and development stage
    2. Clinical research and development stage
    3. New drug application review
    4. Postmarketing surveillance
26. The phase of drug development dealing with the therapeutic value and whether the drug appears to be safe in animals is known as the: *(7)*
    1. preclinical research and development stage.
    2. clinical research and development stage.
    3. new drug application review.
    4. postmarketing surveillance.

27. The Black Box Warning indicates that a drug that is already FDA-approved may have an: *(8)*
    1. associated risk of causing serious or life-threatening adverse effects.
    2. extremely high cost.
    3. effect that may cause nausea and vomiting.
    4. equally effective alternative drug.

Differentiate between the Canadian *chemical* name and the *proper* name of a drug.

28. The nurse is discussing the names of drugs with a patient in Canada, explaining that the difference between the chemical drug name and the proper name is that the: *(9)*
    1. chemical name identifies the manufacturer.
    2. proper name of the drug is also the generic name of the drug.
    3. proper name is most meaningful to the patient.
    4. chemical name identifies the drug as recreational.
29. The *proprietary* name of a Canadian drug refers to the drug's: *(9)*
    1. generic name.
    2. manufacturer.
    3. classification.
    4. brand name.
30. A nurse was explaining to a patient that the difference between the generic name of the drug and the proper name is: *(9)*
    1. the official name will be difficult to pronounce.
    2. generally, there is no difference between the two names.
    3. the proper name is easy to remember.
    4. the proper name is usually the generic name of the drug.

Basic Principles of Drug Action and Drug Interactions

chapter
2

Answer Key: Textbook page references are provided as a guide for answering these questions. A complete answer key is provided to your instructor.

MATCHING
Match the route of administration on the right with the medication on the left. Routes will be used more than once.

Medications

1. _____ oral acetaminophen (Tylenol)
2. _____ subcutaneous insulin (Aspart)
3. _____ intravenous furosemide (Lasix)
4. _____ albuterol (Ventolin) nebulizer
5. _____ sublingual ondansetron (Zofran)

Route of Administration

a. percutaneous
b. enteral
c. parenteral

REVIEW QUESTIONS

Identify common drug administration routes.

6. The nurse knows that drugs are administered by which three most common routes? *(Select all that apply.)* **(14)**
   1. Enteral
   2. Distribution
   3. Percutaneous
   4. Parenteral
   5. Liberation
7. The enteral route includes medications administered: **(14)**
   1. subcutaneously.
   2. orally.
   3. transdermally.
   4. intravenously.
8. The nurse is explaining to the patient that the drug insulin given as a subcutaneous injection is best absorbed: **(14)**
   1. after the patient has eaten a meal.
   2. when deposited into the correct tissue.
   3. if the peripheral circulation is impaired.
   4. when a lump remains at the site of injection.

Identify the meaning and significance of the term *half-life* when used in relation to drug therapy.

9. A measure of the time required for elimination of a drug from the body is known as the: **(15)**
   1. expiration time.
   2. minimum life.
   3. circulation time.
   4. half-life.
10. The nurse knows that the drug alprazolam (Xanax) has a half-life of 12 hours, which means that how much drug will be left circulating in the body after 24 hours? **(16)**
    1. 50%
    2. 30%
    3. 25%
    4. 15%
11. The half-life of a drug may become considerably longer in patients who have which condition(s)? *(Select all that apply.)* **(16)**
    1. Impaired kidney function
    2. Decreased thyroid function
    3. Impaired immune function
    4. Impaired liver function
    5. Decreased amounts of hemoglobin

Describe the process of how a drug is metabolized in the body.

12. List in order the five stages that all drugs go through after they have been administered. *(14)*
    1. _____ Metabolism
    2. _____ Distribution
    3. _____ Excretion
    4. _____ Liberation
    5. _____ Absorption

13. How fast drugs are transferred from the site of entry into the body to the circulation depends on which factor(s)? *(Select all that apply.)* *(14)*
    1. Adequate amounts of fluid (usually water) when given orally
    2. Deposited into the correct tissue when given parenterally
    3. A lump remains at the injection site when given subcutaneously
    4. Reconstituted with the correct diluent recommended by the manufacturer
    5. How fine the droplet particles are for inhaled drugs

14. Drugs are rapidly dispersed throughout the body when administered by which route? *(15)*
    1. Oral
    2. Subcutaneous
    3. Intravenous
    4. Topical

Compare and contrast the following terms that are used in relationship to medications: *desired action*, *common adverse effects*, *serious adverse effects*, *allergic reactions*, and *idiosyncratic reactions*.

15. What is meant by a *desired* drug action? *(17)*
    1. The predictable/usual response to the drug
    2. An unusual or idiosyncratic response to a drug
    3. A response capable of inducing cell mutations
    4. The unpredictable/unusual response to the drug

16. The nurse notices that the patient frequently complains about feeling queasy after taking her morning medications. What is the term for this response ? *(17)*
    1. The desired effect
    2. A serious adverse effect
    3. A common adverse effect
    4. An idiosyncratic reaction

17. Patients who have allergic reactions from an administered drug typically experience which signs/symptoms? *(Select all that apply.)* *(18)*
    1. Severe itching
    2. Hives
    3. Diarrhea
    4. Respiratory distress
    5. Abdominal pain

18. A nurse caring for a patient who was hospitalized after developing thrombocytopenia (low platelets) from taking a prescribed medication knows this response is called: *(17)*
    1. the desired drug effect.
    2. an adverse drug effect.
    3. an allergic reaction.
    4. an idiosyncratic reaction.

19. A patient asked the nurse what the healthcare provider meant by calling his current symptoms *idiosyncratic*. What would be an appropriate response by the nurse? *(18)*
    1. "Your reaction to the medication is really just an allergy."
    2. "The reaction you had to the medication was not what we expected from the drug."
    3. "Your reaction to the drug is typical of what we see from people who have this condition."
    4. "You have had a severe reaction to the medication you are taking and we need to switch your medication."

Identify what is meant by a *drug interaction*.

20. When are drug interactions said to occur? *(Select all that apply.)* *(18)*
    1. Interactions occur when one drug increases the action of one or both drugs.
    2. Interactions occur when one drug inhibits the absorption of another.
    3. Interactions occur when drugs are administered 2 hours apart.
    4. Interactions occur when the effectiveness of one drug or both drugs is decreased.
    5. Interactions occur when drugs cause living cells to mutate.

21. When is a drug considered pharmacologically active? *(15)*
    1. When the drug is bound to plasma proteins
    2. When the drug is unbound from plasma proteins
    3. When the drug is distributed evenly throughout the body
    4. When the drug is metabolized by the liver

22. What resources can the nurse use to aid in determining when a drug interaction will occur? *(Select all that apply.)* *(18)*
    1. Consult with the pharmacist.
    2. Look up possible reactions in drug reference books.
    3. Ask the patient when he or she expects the drugs to interact.
    4. Memorize all possible drug interactions.
    5. Administer each drug several hours apart to ensure nothing happens.

Differentiate among the terms *additive effect,*
synergistic effect, antagonistic effect, displacement,
interference, **and** *incompatibility.*

23. What is the term for when a combination of two
    drugs provides a greater effect than the sum of the
    effect of each drug given alone? *(19)*
    1. Additive effect
    2. Antagonistic effect
    3. Synergistic effect
    4. Displacement effect
24. What is the term for the effect of one drug interfer-
    ing with the effect of another drug? *(19)*
    1. Additive effect
    2. Synergistic effect
    3. Antagonistic effect
    4. Displacement effect
25. What is the name of a common drug interaction
    that inhibits the metabolism or excretion of a second
    drug, thereby causing increased activity of the sec-
    ond drug? *(19)*
    1. Interference
    2. Incompatibility
    3. Antagonistic effect
    4. Additive effect
26. What is the term for when two drugs that have simi-
    lar action are taken for an increased effect? *(19)*
    1. Antagonistic effect
    2. Displacement effect
    3. Synergistic effect
    4. Additive effect
27. The drugs ampicillin and gentamicin are said to be
    incompatible because they cause what effect? *(19)*
    1. The ampicillin displaces gentamicin from
       protein-binding sites.
    2. The ampicillin inactivates gentamicin.
    3. The ampicillin inhibits the excretion of gentami-
       cin.
    4. The ampicillin induces enzymes to metabolize
       gentamicin.

28. The term *displacement* refers to the drug-drug inter-
    action that causes the first drug to have what effect
    on the second drug? *(19)*
    1. The first drug inhibits the metabolism of the
       second drug.
    2. The first drug becomes unbound by the second
       drug, increasing its effect.
    3. The first drug increases the effect of the second
       drug.
    4. The first drug decreases the half-life of the sec-
       ond drug.

Identify one way in which alternatives in metabolism
create drug interactions.

29. What occurs as a result of inhibition of enzymes that
    metabolize drugs? *(18)*
    1. There is an increase in drug interactions.
    2. There are more incompatibility issues.
    3. There is an increase in protein-bound drugs.
    4. There is a decrease in absorption rates.
30. When the metabolism of a drug is inhibited, then
    serum drug levels increase and may lead to what
    effect? *(18)*
    1. Increased displacement
    2. Increased bound drugs
    3. Accumulation and toxicity
    4. Drug incompatibility
31. How should the dosage of a drug such as rifampin,
    which binds to an enzyme that increases its metabo-
    lism (an enzyme inducer), be adjusted? *(19)*
    1. Generally decreased
    2. Generally increased
    3. Remain at the same dose
    4. Discontinued

Drug Action Across the Life Span

Answer Key: Textbook page references are provided as a guide for answering these questions. A complete answer key is provided to your instructor.

Matching

Match the correct definition of a drug action with the key term.

Key Term

1. _____ placebo
2. _____ tolerance
3. _____ polypharmacy
4. _____ protein binding
5. _____ teratogens

Definition of a Drug Action

a. the use of multiple drugs for chronic illness that increases risk of drug interactions
b. drugs that cause birth defects
c. how drugs are circulated in the blood
d. a drug form that has no active ingredients
e. when a person needs a higher dose to produce the same effect

REVIEW QUESTIONS

Explain the impact of the placebo effect and nocebo effect.

6. The nurse is explaining to a patient who is entering into a research study that he may actually get a placebo. Which statement by the patient indicates an understanding of the placebo effect? *(23)*
   1. "I will get the drug that they are testing for my condition."
   2. "I could possibly get a pill that will have a negative effect on my condition."
   3. "The placebo is a drug that has no active ingredients."
   4. "The placebo will have the same effect as the real drug."
7. What is the difference between the placebo effect and the nocebo effect? *(Select all that apply.) (23)*
   1. The nocebo effect has occurred because the patient had negative expectations about the therapy.
   2. The placebo effect has occurred because the patient had negative expectations about the therapy.
   3. The nocebo effect has occurred because the patient had positive expectations about the therapy.
   4. The placebo effect has occurred because the patient had positive expectations about the therapy.
   5. The nocebo effect has occurred because the patient had no particular expectations about the therapy.

8. The attitudes and expectations of the patient regarding the treatment of his or her condition play a major role in a patient's response to therapy. What does the nurse understand this to mean? *(23)*
   1. That patients with chronic silent conditions such as hypertension are more likely to adhere to the prescribed therapy.
   2. That patients with conditions such as arthritis are least likely to adhere to the therapy prescribed.
   3. That patients with conditions that have rapid consequences if therapy is not followed are more likely to adhere to the prescribed therapy.
   4. That patients who had previous negative experiences are more likely to adhere to the prescribed therapy.

Identify the importance of drug dependence and drug accumulation.

9. When does drug dependence occur most often in patients? *(23)*
   1. When patients are unable to ingest drugs.
   2. When patients have indicated they have adequate pain relief from opioids.
   3. When patients are considered incompetent to make any medical decisions.
   4. When patients develop withdrawal symptoms if the drug is discontinued.

10. What patient action could cause the nurse to suspect that the patient has become dependent on the drug oxycodone? *(23)*
    1. The patient is asking for pain medicine more frequently than prescribed.
    2. The patient has become groggy and hard to arouse about an hour after his dose.
    3. The patient is indicating that there is adequate pain relief with the dose.
    4. The patient is worried about becoming addicted to oxycodone and therefore will not take it.

11. When a patient becomes groggy and hard to arouse after receiving a dose of morphine, the patient may be experiencing which drug effect? *(23)*
    1. Dependence
    2. Tolerance
    3. Accumulation
    4. Withdrawal

Discuss the effects of age on drug absorption, distribution, metabolism, and excretion.

12. In relation to drugs and the aging process, the nurse knows which is true? *(24-25)*
    1. Drugs have the same rate of absorption, distribution, metabolism, and excretion as people age.
    2. Drugs will have the same rate of absorption as people age, but their excretion will be affected by changes in the kidneys.
    3. The liver will increase its ability to metabolize drugs as people age.
    4. Pathologic conditions may alter the rate of drug absorption, distribution, metabolism, and excretion.

13. When administering drugs to children, what is important for the nurse to remember? *(23-24)*
    1. Oral tablets are the easiest dose form to administer to children.
    2. Subcutaneous injections will be the most dangerous drug route to administer to children.
    3. Transdermal drug doses are the most difficult route of administration for children.
    4. Liquid medications are the easiest dose form to administer to children.

14. Crushing medications is often done for ease of administration to older adults, and is considered safe when giving which form of medication? *(29)*
    1. Enteric-coated tablets
    2. Sublingual tablets
    3. Tablet and capsule forms
    4. Timed-release tablets

Explain the gender-specific considerations of drug absorption, distribution, metabolism, and excretion.

15. Drug absorption is influenced by which difference in men and women? *(Select all that apply.) (24)*
    1. The difference in gastric motility.
    2. The difference in gastric emptying time.
    3. The different enzyme activity (cytochrome P450) between men and women.
    4. The difference in saliva production.
    5. The difference in gastric pH.

16. Drug distribution is influenced by the difference in men and women's: *(Select all that apply.) (24-25)*
    1. quantity of fat tissue.
    2. protein binding.
    3. gastric emptying time.
    4. cardiac output.
    5. regional blood flow to the target organ.

17. Drug metabolism is influenced by the difference in men's and women's: *(Select all that apply.) (26)*
    1. hereditary characteristics or genes.
    2. number of active receptor sites.
    3. ages.
    4. general health.
    5. maturity of the enzyme systems.

18. Drug excretion is influenced by the difference in men's and women's: *(Select all that apply.) (26)*
    1. renal tubule function.
    2. evaporation of the drug through the skin.
    3. exhalation of the drug from the lungs.
    4. fat distribution in the body.
    5. GI tract motility.

19. What recent new rules instituted by the FDA address the use of drugs during pregnancy and breastfeeding? *(31-32)*
    1. New labeling went into effect for drugs approved since 2001.
    2. New drugs need to be formatted differently for use during pregnancy.
    3. New studies need to be done on drugs known to be teratogenic.
    4. New categories are used for drugs that are approved in pregnancy.

Describe where a nurse will find new information about use of drugs during pregnancy and lactation.

20. A new nurse was talking with a seasoned nurse about changes in drug labeling, and the seasoned nurse mentioned that the pregnancy categories have changed. He suggested the new nurse look up the new information on which websites? *(Select all that apply.) (32)*
    1. e-Pocrates
    2. Lexi-Comp
    3. LactMed
    4. HealthNet
    5. DART

21. Databases such as Toxnet were developed for healthcare providers to access what? *(32)*
    1. Information on drugs associated with increased risk to nursing infants
    2. The site to refer patients for more information regarding safe medications during pregnancy
    3. The animal studies that are conducted on medications to determine safety issues
    4. The database for journals covering teratology and reproductive toxicology
22. Which online resource for healthcare providers includes information on drugs during pregnancy and lactation? *(32)*
    1. DailyMed
    2. NANDA
    3. DART
    4. MedMD

Discuss the impact of pregnancy and breastfeeding on drug absorption, distribution, metabolism, and excretion.

23. The nurse knows that a nursing mother has been taking paroxetine (Paxil) and has explained to her that taking this drug will have what effect? *(32)*
    1. The drug will interfere with the metabolism of a nursing infant.
    2. The drug is associated with significant effects on nursing infants.
    3. The drug has an unknown effect, but may be of concern for a nursing infant.
    4. The drug is reported to have adverse effects on nursing infants.
24. It is safe to take medications during pregnancy and while breastfeeding if the drug is: *(31)*
    1. an herbal product.
    2. labeled by the FDA as safe.
    3. known to be teratogenic.
    4. nonprescription only.

25. What general principle can be applied to pregnant women with regard to drug therapy? *(31)*
    1. No drugs are safe during pregnancy.
    2. All drugs are safe during pregnancy.
    3. Only drugs that have been approved by the FDA are safe during pregnancy.
    4. All herbal products have been determined as safe during pregnancy.

Discuss the role of genetics and its influence on drug action.

26. *Genetics* refers to the study of how living organisms inherit the characteristics or traits of their ancestors and include which characteristics? *(Select all that apply.)* *(33)*
    1. Hair color
    2. Body build
    3. Food preferences
    4. Skin pigmentation
    5. Parenting style
27. Why is the Human Genome Project important for biomedical research? *(33)*
    1. Because the project will help predict when a person will get sick.
    2. The genome will help researchers study the side effect profiles of different medications.
    3. Because the project can now determine what causes cancer.
    4. The genome determines which chromosome was inherited from the mother and which from the father.
28. Why are genetic polymorphisms important in pharmacology? *(33)*
    1. Because they eliminate drug interactions or drug toxicity.
    2. Because they will impact drug metabolism and excretion.
    3. Because they tend to become teratogenic.
    4. Because they decrease the need for drugs.

The Nursing Process and Pharmacology

Answer Key: Textbook page references are provided as a guide for answering these questions. A complete answer key is provided to your instructor.

MATCHING

Match the type of nursing action on the right with the example of nursing action on the left. Types will be used more than once.

Example of Nursing Action

1. _____ reviewing a medication prescription
2. _____ determining when to turn a patient in bed
3. _____ obtaining the patient's medication history
4. _____ collaborating with the prescriber when to give a medication
5. _____ formulating an appropriate nursing diagnosis
6. _____ determining the frequency of drug administration

Type of Nursing Action

a. independent nursing action
b. interdependent nursing action
c. dependent nursing action

REVIEW QUESTIONS

Discuss the components and purpose of the nursing process.

7. Nurses use the nursing process to: *(36)*
   1. build a framework for consistent nursing actions.
   2. assign nursing staff to patients.
   3. standardize the language nurses use to analyze nursing care.
   4. solve problems in nursing systematically.
8. An important aspect of the nursing process is that it uses which approach? *(36)*
   1. Intuitive
   2. Problem-solving
   3. Scientific
   4. Analytical
9. List in order the steps used in the nursing process: *(37)*
   1. _____ Nursing diagnosis
   2. _____ Evaluation
   3. _____ Assessment
   4. _____ Planning
   5. _____ Implementation

10. The nurse considers the patient's psychosocial and cultural needs during which step of the nursing process? *(37)*
    1. Assessment
    2. Planning
    3. Nursing diagnosis
    4. Implementation
11. The nurse uses which step of the nursing process to detect any potential complications? *(38)*
    1. Assessment
    2. Planning
    3. Nursing diagnosis
    4. Implementation

Explain what the nurse does to collect patient information during an assessment.

12. Nurses perform the task of patient assessment to determine: *(Select all that apply.)* *(39)*
    1. the patient's response to treatments.
    2. any adverse effects of medications.
    3. the status of their discharge plans.
    4. if the medical diagnosis is correct.
    5. if the patient has any risk factors.

13. The initial assessment is performed on a patient to identify patient problems based on defining characteristics, as well as to identify: *(Select all that apply.)* *(39)*
    1. any risk factors that predispose the patient to developing problems.
    2. the patient's response to their disease process.
    3. any adverse effects of medications.
    4. when the patient needs assistance to get up in the chair.
    5. what to prescribe for treatment for various disease processes.
14. Important healthcare information that the nurse gathers during the assessment of a patient includes which component(s)? *(Select all that apply.)* *(39)*
    1. vital signs
    2. lung sounds
    3. mobility level
    4. discharge plans
    5. family support
15. Gordon's Functional Health Patterns model is an example of what kind of assessment? *(39)*
    1. Body systems approach
    2. Head-to-toe approach
    3. Sociocultural, psychological, spiritual, and developmental approach
    4. High-risk signs and symptoms approach
16. The nurse needs to assess the patient in the hospital for therapeutic effects, side effects, and potential drug interactions during which time? *(39)*
    1. Throughout the hospitalization
    2. When the patient has visitors
    3. When the patient requests a PRN medication
    4. While monitoring vital signs

Discuss how nursing diagnosis statements are written.

17. What does NANDA stand for when referring to nursing diagnoses? *(39)*
    1. Not All Nursing Diagnosis Association
    2. Natural Accented Northern Diagnosis Adaptable
    3. Nursing Accountable Nursing Diagnosis Authority
    4. North American Nursing Diagnosis Association
18. NANDA diagnoses are part of the nursing language that describes which types of diagnoses? *(Select all that apply.)* *(39)*
    1. Syndrome nursing diagnoses
    2. Actual medical diagnoses
    3. Risk/high-risk nursing diagnoses
    4. Wellness nursing diagnoses
    5. Health promotion diagnoses

19. When writing the outcome statement for medication therapy, the nurse will describe the expected outcomes from the prescribed medications based on what? *(43)*
    1. The etiology and contributing factors involved
    2. The patient's laboratory test results
    3. The recommended routes of the medications
    4. The noted improvement of the symptoms present.

Differentiate between a nursing diagnosis and a medical diagnosis.

20. The nurse analyzes the data collected from the patient assessment to identify signs and symptoms that will be addressed under the nursing diagnosis. These are known as the: *(41)*
    1. therapeutic intent.
    2. defining characteristics.
    3. measurable outcomes.
    4. contributing factors.
21. When formulating the nursing diagnosis in relation to medications, the nurse will need to identify problems related to medication therapy and should review the: *(45)*
    1. medical diagnosis.
    2. drug monographs.
    3. therapeutic responses.
    4. procedures to ensure patient safety.
22. Which two types of nursing diagnoses apply to all types of medication therapies? *(45)*
    1. Deficient knowledge and Deficient diversional activity
    2. Noncompliance and Deficient knowledge
    3. Risk-prone health behavior and Noncompliance
    4. Deficient knowledge and Interrupted family processes
23. How do nursing diagnoses differ from medical diagnoses? *(40)*
    1. The medical diagnosis identifies defining characteristics.
    2. The nursing diagnosis identifies alterations in structure and function.
    3. The medical diagnosis identifies alterations in structure and function.
    4. The nursing diagnosis identifies a disease or disorder that impairs function.
24. What are the three components of the nursing diagnosis? *(41)*
    1. Defining characteristics, identified disease processes, and contributing factors
    2. Alterations in function, NANDA-approved label, and identified disease process
    3. Defining characteristics, contributing factors, and etiology of the disorder
    4. NANDA-approved label, defining characteristics, and contributing factors

Discuss how evidence-based practice is used in planning nursing care.

25. When nurses use evidence-based practice changes for planning nursing care, they are incorporating what factor into the nursing process? *(41)*
    1. Traditional expectations
    2. Trial and error
    3. Pilot studies
    4. Validated research

26. The goal of evidence-based practice is to improve patient outcomes by using what? *(41)*
    1. Various treatments for medical conditions
    2. Best practices that evolved from research
    3. The patient's clinical presentation
    4. Prescriptive recommendations of healthcare providers

27. Discontinuing the use of antiembolism stockings because recent studies have shown them to be ineffective is an example of: *(41)*
    1. nursing intuition.
    2. trial and error.
    3. evidence-based nursing practice.
    4. traditional nursing practice.

28. Which four phases are included in the process used for planning patient interventions? *(Select all that apply.) (41)*
    1. The nurse sets priorities.
    2. The nurse develops measurable goals.
    3. The nurse identifies "related to" factors.
    4. The nurse formulates nursing interventions.
    5. The nurse formulates therapeutic outcomes.

Differentiate between nursing interventions and expected outcome statements.

29. Nursing interventions identify specific nursing actions, while measurable goal statements identify specific: *(42)*
    1. priority settings.
    2. patient behaviors.
    3. changes in patient care needs.
    4. patient responses.

30. Why is it important for nurses to include the patient and appropriate significant others in decision-making when formulating therapeutic patient outcomes? *(43)*
    1. Because it will help promote cooperation and compliance by the patient
    2. Because it will help provide patients with a sense of control over their care
    3. Because it will help prepare the patient for evidence-based nursing care
    4. Because it will help promote shorter hospital stays

31. How will the nurse identify the therapeutic outcomes of the medications during the planning phase of the nursing process? *(Select all that apply.) (45-46)*
    1. By reviewing the drug monograph for common and serious adverse effects
    2. By filling out an insurance claim for reimbursement
    3. By identifying the therapeutic intent of the medications
    4. By educating the patient how to self-administer medications
    5. By identifying the recommended dosage of the medications

Explain how Maslow's hierarchy of needs is used to prioritize patient needs.

32. When is Maslow's hierarchy of human needs used in the planning process? *(42)*
    1. When setting priorities
    2. When developing measurable goals
    3. When formulating therapeutic outcomes
    4. When identifying "related to" factors

33. The five levels of needs identified by Maslow's hierarchy include: *(Select all that apply.) (42)*
    1. self-actualization.
    2. safety.
    3. belonging.
    4. physiologic.
    5. priority.

34. Which level of Maslow's hierarchy would be a priority when planning nursing care? *(42)*
    1. Safety needs
    2. Belonging needs
    3. Self-esteem needs
    4. Physiologic needs

Compare and contrast the differences among dependent, interdependent, and independent nursing actions.

35. The nurse is performing a *dependent* nursing action in which scenario? *(43)*
    1. The patient is being monitored for the effects of the medication given at 8 AM.
    2. The patient is being educated on her 8 AM medication by the nurse.
    3. The patient is given her 8 AM medication by the nurse.
    4. The patient is verbalizing that she understands the reasons for the medications she received at 8 AM.

36. The nurse is performing an *interdependent* nursing action in which scenario? *(43)*
    1. The nurse is calling the healthcare provider for pain medication prescriptions.
    2. The nurse is assisting the physical therapist with exercises for the patient.
    3. The nurse is assessing the patient for bowel sounds after surgery.
    4. The nurse is educating the patient in the use of her incentive spirometer.
37. The nurse is performing an *independent* nursing action in which scenarios? *(Select all that apply.)* *(43)*
    1. The patient is being monitored for the effects of the medication given at 8 AM.
    2. The nurse is calling the provider for pain medication prescriptions.
    3. The nurse is educating the patient in the use of the incentive spirometer.
    4. The nurse is assessing the patient for bowel sounds after surgery.
    5. The nurse is consulting with dietary services for patient preference for meals.

Discuss how the nursing process applies to pharmacology.

38. What are the sources that the nurse uses to obtain a medication history? *(Select all that apply.)* *(44-45)*
    1. Objective data (observed by the nurse)
    2. Other healthcare professionals
    3. Subjective data (provided by the patient)
    4. Drug monographs
    5. The electronic medical record

39. When discussing the medication history with a patient, the nurse will ask the patient to identify current medications and drug allergies, as well as what other important factor(s)? *(Select all that apply.)* *(44)*
    1. Any diagnostic tests done
    2. Any over-the-counter medications used
    3. Any food allergies
    4. Any herbal products used
    5. Any street drugs used
40. The nurse can use primary, secondary, and tertiary sources to gain information to complete the medication history. When the nurse obtains vital signs to use as monitoring parameters later, it is considered which source of information? *(44)*
    1. A secondary source of information
    2. A tertiary source of information
    3. A primary source of subjective data
    4. A primary source of objective data
41. The medication history that the nurse records includes which important facts to note? *(44)*
    1. Current medications being taken by the patient and drug allergies
    2. Past medications that are no longer being used and drug allergies
    3. Medications that are prescription-based and drug allergies
    4. Over-the-counter medications and drug allergies

Student Name_____ Date_____

Patient Education to Promote Health

Answer Key: Textbook page references are provided as a guide for answering these questions. A complete answer key is provided to your instructor.

MATCHING

Match the learning domain on the right with the patient education objective on the left. Domains may be used more than once.

Patient Education Objective

1. _____ demonstrating correct self-administration of insulin
2. _____ requesting more information on adverse effects of a new medication
3. _____ discussing healthcare changes that will occur when discharged, like needing an aide
4. _____ verbalizing the medications needed for pain relief after surgery

Learning Domain

a. cognitive domain
b. affective domain
c. psychomotor domain

REVIEW QUESTIONS

Differentiate among cognitive, affective, and psychomotor learning domains.

5. When the nurse asks the patient to perform a return demonstration of a skill such as injecting insulin or performing a dressing change, the patient is exercising which domain of learning? *(51)*
   1. Affective
   2. Psychomotor
   3. Cognitive
   4. Psychological
6. The *affective* domain of learning refers to: *(50)*
   1. the thinking portion of the learning process.
   2. learning a new procedure or skill.
   3. feelings, beliefs, and values that the patient has.
   4. the environment that is conducive to learning.
7. The patient has just been instructed on his home-going medications prior to discharge, and the nurse will validate the information that was given by asking the patient to verbalize his understanding. This involves which domain of learning? *(50)*
   1. Cognitive
   2. Affective
   3. Psychomotor
   4. Psychological

Identify the main principles of learning that are applied when teaching a patient, family, or group.

8. When teaching patients and their families, the nurse must recognize the teachable moment when what occurs? *(51)*
   1. The nurse starts to ask questions regarding home-going care.
   2. The nurse has the time and is ready to start teaching the patient.
   3. The patient is gone for a test and the family looks anxious.
   4. The patient starts to ask questions about what to expect when at home.
9. One of the main principles of learning that the nurse incorporates into teaching is that adults learn by: *(51)*
   1. rote memorization.
   2. applying new knowledge to previous learning.
   3. listening to the nurse explain everything.
   4. asking questions.

10. The nurse needs to determine the patient's preferred learning style when educating the patient on continuing care. One way to do this is by using a variety of teaching aids, which may include: *(Select all that apply.)* *(51)*
    1. pamphlets and charts.
    2. discussing care with the family while the patient is out.
    3. DVDs and videos.
    4. smart devices and computer-aided instruction.
    5. filling out the nursing care plan and informing the next shift about it.

Describe the essential elements of patient education in relation to prescribed medications.

11. When the nurse is teaching the patient about medications, which important considerations can be implemented? *(Select all that apply.)* *(51)*
    1. teaching at a time most convenient for the nurse
    2. determining the patient's readiness to learn
    3. spacing the content over several short sessions
    4. organizing the patient education materials
    5. using repetition to enhance learning

12. During a teaching session, the patient suddenly became tearful and turned away. What would be the best response from the nurse at this time? *(52)*
    1. "Why don't you just read this later, and I can mark you as getting through the material."
    2. "I need to finish this and get it checked off my list, so bear with me."
    3. "I see that you are upset; I can finish this later. Do you want to talk about it?"
    4. "I see that you are not paying attention. Now come on, let's finish this."

13. When teaching older adults about new medications, what is important for the nurse to remember? *(Select all that apply.)* *(54)*
    1. Check the patient for vision or hearing aids.
    2. Determine any memory impairment.
    3. Evaluate the gross motor ability of the patient.
    4. Review the content to be covered rapidly.
    5. Lecture the patient about healthy lifestyles.

Describe the nurse's role in fostering patient responsibility for maintaining well-being and for adhering to the therapeutic regimen.

14. The nurse understands that when teaching a patient and family about lifestyle changes, it is important to: *(Select all that apply.)* *(56)*
    1. tell the patient that she will need to change her lifestyle or else.
    2. keep the content of the information relevant to the patient.
    3. add extra content to further explain points.
    4. remember that learning new ideas may be overwhelming.
    5. keep the patient's wishes in mind.

15. What is one important aspect of the nurse's role in discussing the patient's medications and adhering to a particular medication regimen? *(55)*
    1. To adopt a slower pace for teaching younger patients
    2. To dictate to the older adult patient what must be changed
    3. To continue teaching until all content is covered
    4. To repeat the information often, and stop and allow practice

16. The nurse needs to involve the patient in cooperative goal-setting when teaching, which will include discussing what with the patient? *(Select all that apply.)* *(56)*
    1. What the patient should monitor
    2. Why the prescribed therapy is needed
    3. When to call the healthcare provider
    4. Where to collect and record essential data
    5. How to discontinue or alter their medication regimen

Identify the types of information that should be discussed with the patient or significant others.

17. The nurse is reviewing sources of patient information on the Internet that may be helpful for patients wanting more information after discharge. These sources may include which websites? *(Select all that apply.)* *(56)*
    1. Krames Online
    2. Therapeutic Choices
    3. Health on the Net Foundation
    4. Medline
    5. CINAHL

18. Nurses who tend to be ethnocentric consider patients in light of what? *(55)*
    1. Culture the patient is from
    2. Culture the nurse is from
    3. Hospital the patient is in
    4. Home environment the patient lives in

19. Reasonable expectations that the nurse should have when discussing new treatment therapies include which factor? *(57)*
    1. That the patient will fully understand all instructions
    2. That the patient and family will ask appropriate questions and demonstrate adequate understanding of teaching
    3. That the family will have participated in the teaching because most patients are unable to think clearly while in the hospital
    4. That the patient will need to be taken care of outside of the hospital, since the instructions will never be understood

Discuss specific techniques used in the practice setting to facilitate patient education.

20. How can the nurse can facilitate appropriate patient teaching? *(57)*
    1. Keep all records of the essential data needed to evaluate the prescribed therapy.
    2. Expect the patient to manage his therapy without further assistance.
    3. Contact the healthcare provider for advice on when to tell the patient to discontinue his medication entirely.
    4. Ask the patient to record responses to his medications at home.

21. Which statement by a patient indicates that further teaching is needed? *(57)*
    1. "I will keep a record of my blood pressure the same time of day to see how my medication is working."
    2. "I know that I will need to call my healthcare provider when I start to feel like I did when I came into the hospital."
    3. "I can take my pills when I feel like it, because they can get so expensive."
    4. "I will let my wife know about these pills because she usually helps me remember to take them."

22. When a patient is discharged from the hospital, what is important for the nurse to document? *(58)*
    1. The time the patient left and who accompanied the patient
    2. All care that was received during hospitalization
    3. The collaborative problems that will require continued monitoring after discharge
    4. The nursing diagnoses that were identified on admission

Principles of Medication Administration and Medication Safety

Answer Key: Textbook page references are provided as a guide for answering these questions. A complete answer key is provided to your instructor.

MATCHING
Match the rights of drug administration on the right with the nursing action on the left. Rights may be used more than once.

Nursing Action

1. _____ triple-check the drug
2. _____ consult reference book and calculate properly
3. _____ verify the reason for the drug
4. _____ this affects absorption rate
5. _____ check to determine when drug was given last
6. _____ compare exact spelling
7. _____ a major medicolegal consideration
8. _____ ensure two identifiers are used
9. _____ determine appropriate schedule

Seven Rights of Drug Administration

a. right drug
b. right indication
c. right time
d. right dose
e. right patient
f. right route
g. right documentation

REVIEW QUESTIONS

Identify the legal and ethical considerations for medication administration.

10. The rules and regulations established by the state boards of nursing are in place to ensure what? *(61)*
    1. That there are guidelines in place to practice nursing
    2. To restrict access to healthcare
    3. What will be done when an avoidable complication arises
    4. To regulate healthcare facilities
11. Policy statements that are made by nurse practice acts related to medication administration include: *(Select all that apply.) (61)*
    1. educational requirements necessary to have prescriptive privileges.
    2. lists of medications that are forbidden to be administered by nurses.
    3. abbreviations approved for use to avoid medication errors.
    4. medications that the nurse can start with IV solutions.
    5. when to claim unfamiliarity with any nursing responsibilities.

12. Prior to any medication administration, the nurse must be able to do what? *(Select all that apply.) (61)*
    1. Accurately calculate the drug dose
    2. Document the patient's response to the medication
    3. Explain to the patient the expected actions of the medication
    4. Explain to the patient why the medication is prescribed
    5. Describe the contraindications for the use of the medication

Compare and contrast the various systems used to dispense medications.

13. The floor stock system of dispensing medications used in small hospitals has the advantage of readily available medications, but also what disadvantage? *(Select all that apply.)* **(68)**
    1. There is increased potential for medication errors.
    2. There is the potential misappropriation of medication by hospital personnel.
    3. There are fewer inpatient prescription orders.
    4. There is a lack of review by a pharmacist for patient prescription accuracy.
    5. There is a need for larger stocks and frequent drug inventories.

14. Which system used to dispense medications provides the advantage of fewer inpatient prescription orders and minimal return of medications? **(68-69)**
    1. The unit-dose system
    2. The floor or ward stock system
    3. The individual prescription order system
    4. The computer-controlled dispensing system

15. What are advantages of the unit-dose system? **(69)**
    1. Returned bottles of unused medications are destroyed.
    2. There is less waste and misappropriation of medications.
    3. Quality-control procedures are completed by healthcare providers.
    4. Packaging of medications require counting drugs from multidose packets.

16. *Pyxis system* refers to what drug dosage system? **(69)**
    1. Narcotic inventory system
    2. Individual prescription order system
    3. Unit-dose system used primarily in long-term care
    4. Electronic medication dispensing system

17. What does the *ward stock system* refer to? **(68)**
    1. A narcotic inventory system
    2. An individual prescription order system
    3. A system used in very small hospitals
    4. An electronic medication dispensing system

18. The nurse understands that using a computer-controlled ordering and dispensing system means what? **(69-70)**
    1. That there is no need to use standard procedures for medications like the seven rights.
    2. That the verification and transcription of medication prescriptions are built into the system.
    3. The need to account for the narcotic inventory will no longer be necessary.
    4. Documentation of the patient's response to the medication is not needed.

Identify what a narcotic control system entails.

19. When removing narcotics from a narcotic control system, what must be recorded at the time of removal? *(Select all that apply.)* **(71)**
    1. The medications must be passcode-accessible
    2. The name of the patient
    3. The time the medication was removed
    4. The name of the nurse who removed the medication
    5. The time the medication was given to the patient

20. A nurse was preparing to administer 3 mg of morphine (a controlled substance) orally to a patient. The medication came in 4 mg/4 mL. What steps must the nurse take when giving this medication? *(Select all that apply.)* **(71)**
    1. Determine the correct amount to give (3 mL).
    2. Ask another nurse to verify the dose and any wasted medication.
    3. Check the time interval since the last dose was given.
    4. Complete the controlled substance inventory.
    5. Complete the documentation after administration.

21. While checking the narcotics count at the end of a shift, the nurse notes a discrepancy regarding the oral doses of hydromorphone (Dilaudid). What needs to be done next? **(71-72)**
    1. Security needs to be called.
    2. The nurse manager needs to be notified.
    3. The patients' charts need to be reviewed for proper documentation.
    4. An appropriate interval of time must be observed before any narcotics can be removed.

Define the four categories of medication orders.

22. What type of drug prescription indicates that nurses are to administer the medication for a specific number of doses? **(73)**
    1. Stat orders
    2. Verbal orders
    3. Single orders
    4. Standing orders

23. The nurse is reviewing an prescription that states "nifedipine 30 mg SL now." This is an example of what type of order? **(73)**
    1. Stat order
    2. Verbal order
    3. Single order
    4. Standing order

24. When should PRN medications be administered? **(73)**
    1. When the patient asks for some.
    2. When the healthcare provider orders it.
    3. When the appropriate time interval has elapsed.
    4. After the patient asks for it and the nurse determines it can be safely administered.

25. When does the drug prescribed using the term *stat* need to be given? *(73)*
    1. Immediately and one time only.
    2. When the patient asks for it.
    3. Immediately and at scheduled time intervals.
    4. At the next opportunity the nurse has to administer the medication.

Identify common types of medication errors and the actions that can be taken to prevent them.

26. The nurse is preparing to administer a patient's 8 AM medications and notes that the dose for the drug raloxifene (Evista) is only 20 mg and not 40 mg. What will the nurse need to do next? *(74)*
    1. Verify the dosage with the healthcare provider.
    2. Notify the pharmacy that the drug dose is in error.
    3. Administer the medication and report the error.
    4. Refuse to administer all of the patient's medications until the error is corrected.

27. Which type of medication errors could a nurse make when administering a drug? *(Select all that apply.)* *(74)*
    1. Errors of omission (missed dose)
    2. Errors of duplication (extra dose given)
    3. Errors of inventory of the drugs
    4. Errors of formatting the prescription wrong
    5. Errors of wrong time

28. Technology is being used to help prevent medication errors by which methods? *(Select all that apply.)* *(74)*
    1. Robotics to administer medications to free up nurses
    2. System of automatic delivery of medications
    3. Programs that have computerized provider order entry systems
    4. Smart pumps for controlled administration of controlled medications
    5. Barcoded labeling of medications for administration

29. After administering a dose of the oral antihistamine fexofenadine (Allegra), the nurse noticed the patient had already received a dose 2 hours before. What is this type of error called? *(74)*
    1. A prescribing error
    2. An administration error
    3. A monitoring error
    4. A transcription error

30. During the administration of a medication, the patient asks the nurse why the medication has been prescribed. The nurse will respond with which one of the seven rights? *(76)*
    1. Right patient
    2. Right route
    3. Right dosage
    4. Right indication

31. When preparing to administer a medication to a patient, the nurse is not able to verify that the medication prescription is appropriate. What actions does the nurse take? *(Select all that apply.)* *(75-76)*
    1. Contacts the healthcare provider who prescribed the drug
    2. Documents the reasons for refusal to administer the drug in accordance with the policies of the agency
    3. Informs the patient about the disagreement with the treatment prescribed
    4. If the prescriber cannot be contacted, notifies the nursing supervisor on duty
    5. Administers the medication because it went through pharmacy, and they would have caught a problem if there was one

Identify precautions used to ensure the right drug is prepared and given to the right patient.

32. The nurse was preparing to administer a dose of the antibiotic cefepime (Maxipime). Place the steps in the order that the nurse will follow to ensure the right drug is administered. *(76-79)*
    1. _____ Document the drug.
    2. _____ Triple-check that the drug name and dose are correct prior to administration.
    3. _____ Identify the patient using two patient identifiers.
    4. _____ Administer the medication via the correct route.
    5. _____ Check the prescription.

33. Medication reconciliation is a process designed to reduce medication errors and involves which steps? *(Select all that apply.)* *(75)*
    1. Comparing written blanket prescriptions
    2. Reviewing potential adverse drug events
    3. Developing a list of prescribed medications
    4. Developing a list of current medications being taken by the patient
    5. Comparing the lists of current medications with prescribed ones

34. After the patient returns from an elective procedure, the healthcare provider writes a prescription that states, "Resume all preprocedure medications." What is this known as? *(75)*
    1. A handoff order
    2. Medication reconciliation
    3. A blanket order
    4. A redundant order

List the seven rights of medication administration.

35. After the nurse has administered an appropriate dose of a medication that has been prescribed, the nurse must now do what? *(79)*
    1. Scan the medication into the barcode system.
    2. Notify the prescriber that the medication has been administered.
    3. Document in the medication administration record the date and time given.
    4. Review the prescription and perform triple-checks.

36. When reconstituting a medication to be administered, the nurse needs to clearly label it with what? *(Select all that apply.) (78)*
    1. The patient's name
    2. The correct dose
    3. The proper concentration
    4. The amount to be discarded
    5. The name of the drug

37. What is the most effective method the nurse uses for identifying a pediatric patient for medication administration? *(78)*
    1. Asking the child his or her name
    2. Asking a family member the child's name
    3. Checking the child's identification bracelet
    4. Checking the room number with the bed the child is in

Identify the appropriate nursing documentation of medications including the effectiveness of each medication.

38. What does the nurse need to document to identify how effective medications are? *(Select all that apply.)* *(80)*
    1. Questions the family asks about home-going medications
    2. Noting any nausea and vomiting after giving oral medications
    3. Monitoring the patient's vital signs
    4. Checking blood sugar after insulin administration
    5. Specific assessments such as lung sounds

39. What does the nurse need to do when determining the therapeutic effectiveness of a medication? *(79)*
    1. Ask the patient to repeat the name of the medication.
    2. Call the healthcare provider to verify each medication prescribed.
    3. Notify the pharmacist of the patient's response.
    4. Document the patient's response and notify the healthcare provider when appropriate.

40. The nurse gave an antiemetic medication 30 minutes ago and is checking on the patient to determine the effectiveness. Which scenario indicates the medication worked? *(79)*
    1. The patient states that he feels much better and his pain is all gone.
    2. The patient states he feels a lot less nauseated.
    3. The patient states he is starting to feel dizzy and lightheaded.
    4. The patient states that he is feeling weaker and getting chills.

Percutaneous Administration

Answer Key: Textbook page references are provided as a guide for answering these questions. A complete answer key is provided to your instructor.

MATCHING

Match the dose form on the right with the application site on the left. More than one dose form may be used for the application sites.

Application Site

1. _____ ear
2. _____ eye
3. _____ skin
4. _____ mucous membranes
5. _____ buccal cavity

Dose Form

a. powders
b. aqueous solutions
c. transdermal patches
d. creams
e. ointments
f. buccal tablets

REVIEW QUESTIONS

Identify the equipment needed and the techniques used to apply each of the topical forms of medications to the skin.

6. The factors affecting the absorption of topical medications include which? *(Select all that apply.)* *(82)*
   1. The concentration of the medication
   2. The length of time the medication is in contact with the skin
   3. The patient's personal hygiene preferences
   4. The thickness and hydration of the skin
   5. The size and depth of the skin area affected

7. The major advantages of the percutaneous route for medication administration include which? *(Select all that apply.)* *(82)*
   1. This route reduces the spread of infection.
   2. This route decreases systemic adverse effects.
   3. This route improves patient personal hygiene measures.
   4. This route has a long duration of action and reapplication is often not required.
   5. This route allows for limited exposure of the medication to a specific site of application.

8. The percutaneous route of medication administration includes which forms of application? *(Select all that apply.)* *(82)*
   1. Eyedrops
   2. Nasal sprays
   3. Rectal suppositories
   4. Subcutaneous injections
   5. Inhaled nebulized medications

9. Why is it important for the nurse to wear gloves when applying a topical ointment or transdermal patch? *(83)*
   1. To identify a patient's sensitivity to contact materials
   2. So the correct amount of medication is applied to the patient's skin
   3. So the dose is not contaminated with the nurse's skin cells
   4. To avoid inadvertent absorption of the medication by the nurse through the skin

10. List the steps in the order in which the nurse would apply a medicated lotion to a patient. *(83-84)*
    1. _____ Apply lotion firmly but gently by dabbing the surface.
    2. _____ Perform hand hygiene and apply gloves.
    3. _____ Document the application.
    4. _____ Shake the suspension well for a uniform appearance of the lotion.
    5. _____ Clean the area and the equipment used, and make sure that the patient is comfortable.

11. What is important for the nurse to remember when applying ointment to a patient's skin? *(Select all that apply.)* *(83)*
    1. Ointments generally cannot be removed easily with water.
    2. Ointments are semisolid preparations of medicinal substances in an oily base.
    3. Ointments are to be applied directly to the skin or mucous membranes.
    4. Ointments must be reapplied frequently because they are absorbed easily.
    5. The use of ointments helps keep the medication in prolonged contact with the skin.

Describe the purpose of and the procedure used for performing patch testing.

12. The purpose of patch testing is to identify what? *(84)*
    1. When a patient will need an antiemetic
    2. Which antibiotic will be effective against an infection
    3. Which specific sensitivity to an allergen the patient has
    4. Which area of the patient's skin is sensitive to topical ointments

13. The nurse is preparing to apply a patch test to a patient, and the patient asks what he will need to remember after leaving the clinic. Which response by the nurse would be most appropriate? *(86)*
    1. "You will need to call the clinic in 48 hours if you have a reaction."
    2. "You will need to report back to the clinic after a week and we will read the results."
    3. "You will not be able to shower for a week while the patch test is on your back."
    4. "You will need to return to the clinic to have the test read in 48 hours."

14. What areas on the body are commonly used for a patch test? *(Select all that apply.)* *(84)*
    1. Face
    2. Thighs
    3. Back
    4. Neck
    5. Arms

15. What are the symbols commonly used for reading reactions to allergen testing? *(Select all that apply.)* *(85)*
    1. ++ (2+) (2- to 3-mm wheal with flare)
    2. ## (2#) (only erythema noted)
    3. − − − (3−) (no wheal response)
    4. ++++ (4+) (> 5-mm wheal)
    5. +++ (3+) (3- to 5-mm wheal with flare)

16. The nurse is working in an allergy clinic. What should the nurse consider when administering allergy testing to patients? *(Select all that apply.)* *(84-85)*
    1. Documenting "no reaction" at the control site on the patient's chart
    2. Ensuring that emergency equipment is in the immediate area in case of an anaphylactic response
    3. Administering antihistamine and antiinflammatory agents immediately before the test
    4. Positioning the patient so that the surface where the test material is to be applied is horizontal
    5. Cleansing the area where the allergens are to be applied with an alcohol wipe and allowing the area to dry before starting testing

17. In addition to documenting the date, time, drug name, dose, and site of administration of the patch test, the nurse needs to document what other factor? *(86)*
    1. Any signs and symptoms of adverse effects
    2. When the patient bathed or showered last
    3. The number of patch test kits available
    4. When hand hygiene was performed

Identify the equipment needed, the sites and techniques used, and the patient education required when nitroglycerin ointment is prescribed.

18. List in the correct order the steps the nurse will use to administer nitroglycerin ointment. *(86)*
    1. _____ Position patient to expose surface to be used, and remove applicator paper from previous dose.
    2. _____ Apply dose to patient's skin and cover with plastic wrap or tape.
    3. _____ Perform hand hygiene and don gloves.
    4. _____ Gather nitroglycerin ointment, applicator paper, and nonallergenic adhesive tape.
    5. _____ Squeeze proper amount of nitroglycerin ointment onto applicator paper.

19. The nurse is applying a nitroglycerin transdermal disk and expects the disk to be applied how often? *(88)*
    1. Every 12 hours
    2. Every day
    3. Every 7 days
    4. Every 3 days

20. After applying a nitroglycerin transdermal disk, what should the nurse educate the patient about? *(88)*
    1. The number of times the disks can be reused
    2. The documentation needed after application
    3. How and when to apply the disks
    4. To never wear the disks while showering

21. The nurse will identify the expected effectiveness of the nitroglycerin ointment when the patient states what has occurred? *(86)*
    1. Itching and a rash with the drug
    2. An increase in angina attacks
    3. Relief from angina attacks
    4. A severe drop in blood pressure and lightheadedness

22. What should documentation of the application of nitroglycerin ointment include? *(Select all that apply.)* *(87)*
    1. When any family is present in the room
    2. That essential patient education that was reviewed
    3. The signs and symptoms of adverse drug effects
    4. The date, time, dosage, site, route of administration, and nurse's name
    5. The patient assessments such as blood pressure, pulse, and pain relief

23. The nurse was completing the process of administering 1 inch of nitroglycerin ointment to the patient's left chest; proper documentation will include the date and what other information? *(87)*
    1. 0915, nitroglycerin ointment (1") to chest, Nancy Nurse
    2. 0915, 1" nitroglycerin ointment applied to left chest, topical, Nancy Nurse
    3. 0915, nitroglycerin ointment, Nancy Nurse
    4. 0915, 1" nitroglycerin ointment, topical, Nancy Nurse

Identify the equipment needed, the sites and techniques used, and the patient education required when transdermal medication systems are prescribed.

24. What does patient education for transdermal medication systems include? *(Select all that apply.)* *(88)*
    1. When to document the administration of the medication
    2. When it is appropriate to take a shower
    3. What to do when the disk becomes loose
    4. When a drug-free period of time is prescribed
    5. When to discontinue using the medication

25. When administering nitroglycerin percutaneously to a patient, what does the nurse do? *(86)*
    1. Performs hand hygiene and wears gloves
    2. Applies wax paper over the site of the nitroglycerin to enhance absorption of the drug
    3. Ensures that the drug is on the patient 24 hours a day, 7 days a week to avoid complications
    4. Always places the nitroglycerin ointment over the left chest to provide the most effective route of drug delivery to the heart

26. The common sites used for application of any transdermal medication disks include which areas of the body? *(Select all that apply.)* *(86)*
    1. Chest
    2. Face
    3. Flank
    4. Upper arms
    5. Axilla

27. The nurse is reviewing an prescription to administer a topical powder to a patient. What should the nurse know prior to administration? *(89)*
    1. The site of application, the indication for the medication, and the expected effects
    2. The site of application, the common adverse effects of the medication, and the family's expectations
    3. The site of application, the intended purpose of the medication, and the patient's usual sleep pattern
    4. The site of application, the patient's bathing preference, and the expected effects

28. Proper administration of powdered medications includes which technique? *(89)*
    1. Applying the powder to wet skin to allow it to "cake" on
    2. Applying the powder over the area, distributing it evenly and smoothing over the area
    3. Shaking the container prior to administration to evenly distribute the medication
    4. Performing hand hygiene before and after administration; gloves are not necessary

29. What is an important point to consider when administering powdered medication? *(89)*
    1. How long the powder needs to stay on
    2. When to wash the powder off
    3. Where to apply the powder
    4. Which medication will wear off faster

Describe the dose forms, the sites and equipment used, and the techniques for the administration of medications to the mucous membranes.

30. List in order the steps the nurse will take to administer eyedrops. *(90)*
    1. _____ Hold the eyelid open and approach the eye from below with the medication dropper.
    2. _____ Discard gloves, perform hand hygiene, and document.
    3. _____ Position the patient so that the back of the head is firmly supported on a pillow and the face is directed toward the ceiling.
    4. _____ Obtain the prescribed bottle or tube of eye medication.
    5. _____ Perform hand hygiene and don gloves.

31. The proper technique used to administer eyedrops or eye ointment is to ask the patient to look which direction? *(90)*
    1. Down and to the left
    2. Up and over your head
    3. Up and to the right
    4. Down and to the right
32. Medications that can be applied to mucous membranes are available in which dose forms? *(Select all that apply.)* *(89)*
    1. Sublingual tablets
    2. Suppository
    3. Transdermal disc
    4. Dry powder inhaler
    5. Buccal tablets

Compare the techniques that are used to administer eardrops to patients who are less than 3 years old with those that are used for patients who are 3 years and older.

33. When administering eardrops to a child younger than 3 years, the nurse should restrain the child, turn the head to the appropriate side, and gently pull the earlobe in which direction? *(92)*
    1. Downward and back
    2. Downward and forward
    3. Upward and back
    4. Upward and forward
34. The nurse is explaining to the mother of a 2-year-old child how to administer eardrops to her child, and the mother asks if cotton can be placed in the ear after administration. Which response by the nurse would be most appropriate? *(92)*
    1. "Yes, that is recommended. Let me show you how."
    2. "No, that practice is not accepted anymore."
    3. "Yes, we can use a cotton-tipped applicator and insert it as far back as it will go."
    4. "No, the healthcare provider will frown on that."
35. When applying eardrops to a child, the nurse notices that there is a large amount of wax buildup in the ear canal. What will the nurse do next? *(92)*
    1. Administer the medication, as the wax will not be a problem.
    2. Remove the wax with a cotton-tipped applicator prior to administration.
    3. Obtain an order to gently remove wax by irrigating the ear canal prior to administration.
    4. Call the healthcare provider and ask for another route for the medication to be administered.

Describe the purpose, the precautions necessary, and the patient education required for those patients who require medications via inhalation.

36. Which types of medications are available in the oral inhalation dose form? *(Select all that apply.)* *(95)*
    1. Bronchodilators
    2. Fentanyl
    3. Nitroglycerin
    4. Corticosteroids
    5. Allergens
37. Bronchodilators and corticosteroids may be administered by oral inhalation through the mouth using which dose form that is aerosolized and pressurized? *(95)*
    1. Semisolid emulsion
    2. Buccal tablet
    3. Metered-dose inhaler (MDI)
    4. Oral drops/oral spray
38. What does the nurse instruct the patient to do when administering medications via the inhalation route? *(Select all that apply.)* *(95)*
    1. Inhale deeply over 10 seconds after activating the MDI.
    2. Shake the medication canister before using MDIs.
    3. Rinse his or her mouth before using an inhaled corticosteroid.
    4. Blow into the dry powder inhaler (DPI).
    5. Place one end of the extender in the mouth and close the lips around it.

Identify the equipment needed, the site, and the specific techniques required to administer vaginal medications or douches.

39. List in order the steps the nurse takes to administer a vaginal suppository. *(98)*
    1. _____ Perform hand hygiene and don gloves.
    2. _____ Lubricate the gloved index finger and insert the suppository.
    3. _____ Ask the patient to void prior to administration.
    4. _____ Place the patient in the correct position and unwrap a vaginal suppository that has been warmed to room temperature, and lubricate it with a water-soluble lubricant.
    5. _____ Document the administration.
40. In what position should the nurse place a patient who is to be administered a vaginal medication? *(98)*
    1. On the left side
    2. On the back with legs in the air
    3. On the stomach with knees tucked
    4. On the back in the lithotomy position
41. Douching is recommended for which use? *(98)*
    1. When there is a vaginal infection present
    2. As a normal feminine hygiene practice
    3. As an effective method of birth control
    4. After a vaginal suppository has been administered

Enteral Administration

chapter

8

Answer Key: Textbook page references are provided as a guide for answering these questions. A complete answer key is provided to your instructor.

MATCHING

Match the term on the right with the definition on the left.

Definition

1. _____ medication dissolved in a concentrated solution of sugar and water
2. _____ medication dissolved in alcohol and water
3. _____ small, cylindrical gelatin containers that hold dry powder or liquid medication
4. _____ dry powdered medication compressed into small disks
5. _____ liquids with solid insoluble drug particles dispersed solution, requires shaking prior to use
6. _____ flat disks in a sugar base form to dissolve slowly in the mouth
7. _____ dispersion of small droplets of water in oil by means of an emulsifying agent

Term

a. tablet
b. capsule
c. lozenge
d. elixir
e. emulsion
f. syrup
g. suspension

REVIEW QUESTIONS

Describe general principles of administering solid forms of oral medications.

8. The *enteral route* refers to medications administered directly into the gastrointestinal (GI) tract; this includes which route? *(Select all that apply.)* **(101)**
   1. Rectally
   2. Orally
   3. Sublingually
   4. Nasogastric (NG) tube
   5. Percutaneous endoscopic gastrostomy (PEG) or G tube

9. What are the advantages of the oral route of medication administration? *(Select all that apply.)* **(101)**
   1. It is easy to administer medications orally.
   2. This route has a slow absorption rate.
   3. This route is the most economical.
   4. The oral route is the most convenient.
   5. It is easy to retrieve medications orally, if given in error.

10. When administering a solid form of medication to a patient, which procedures does the nurse apply? *(Select all that apply.)* **(106)**
    1. Using a tablet-crushing device for appropriate medications when patients have difficulty swallowing
    2. Having the patient place the medication on the front of the tongue
    3. Encouraging the patient to keep the head back while swallowing
    4. Remaining with the patient while the medication is being taken
    5. Having the patient drink a full glass of water with the medication

Compare the different techniques that are used with a unit-dose distribution system and an electronic controlled distribution system.

11. Which system requires the nurse to use a security access code and password? **(105)**
    1. Electronic controlled system
    2. Medication card system
    3. Unit-dose distribution system
    4. Medication administration record system

12. When distributing medications via the computer-controlled system, what will the nurse need to verify the medication? *(105)*
    1. The medication profile
    2. A medication card
    3. Another nurse to verify the correct dosage
    4. The patient to correctly identify the medication
13. Which system is designed to allow the nurse to hand the medication to the patient and allow him or her to read the package label? *(105)*
    1. Computer-controlled system
    2. Unit-dose system
    3. Medication administration record
    4. Medication card system

Identify general principles used for liquid-form oral medication administration.

14. To read the correct amount of a liquid medication that has been poured into a medicine cup, the nurse reads the meniscus at which point? *(107)*
    1. At the lowest point of the convex curve in the cup
    2. At the highest point of the concave curve in the cup
    3. At the lowest point of the concave curve in the cup
    4. At the highest point of the convex curve in the cup
15. What is the term for small droplets of water in oil or oil in water that are used to mask bitter tastes or provide better solubility to certain drugs? *(103)*
    1. An elixir
    2. A suspension
    3. A syrup
    4. An emulsion
16. When administering a liquid form of an oral medication to an infant, what does the nurse need to confirm? *(108)*
    1. That the infant is alert
    2. That the infant is positioned so that the head is lowered
    3. That the syringe or dropper is at the tip of the infant's tongue
    4. That the medicine is given rapidly to facilitate swallowing of the medicine

Cite the equipment needed, techniques used, and precautions necessary when administering medications via a nasogastric tube.

17. The alternative route of giving medications by NG tube is generally done because the patient has which condition? *(Select all that apply.)* *(108)*
    1. The patient is comatose.
    2. The patient is unable to swallow.
    3. The patient has had back surgery.
    4. The patient has a disorder of the esophagus.
    5. The patient refuses to take medications orally.

18. List in order the proper procedure for administration of a drug via an NG tube. *(110)*
    1. _____ Clamp the tubing at the end of medication administration.
    2. _____ Position the patient upright and check the location of the NG tube.
    3. _____ Flush the tube with 30 mL of water using a larger syringe.
    4. _____ Perform hand hygiene and don gloves.
    5. _____ Document the medication and how the patient tolerated the procedure.
19. Why should the nurse flush the NG tube after administration of enteral formulas? *(Select all that apply.)* *(108)*
    1. To remove the formula from the tubing
    2. To maintain the patency of the tube
    3. To allow better absorption of the formula from the stomach
    4. To ensure the tube stays in position after the feeding
    5. To prevent the formula remaining in the tube from supporting bacterial growth
20. When working with patients receiving intermittent enteral feedings via a gastrostomy tube, which position does the patient need to be in? *(109)*
    1. The lithotomy position
    2. The semi-Fowler's position
    3. The prone position
    4. The supine position

Cite the equipment needed and the technique required when administering rectal suppositories and disposable enemas.

21. What instructions will the nurse give the patient when administering a rectal suppository? *(112)*
    1. "Hold your breath while I insert the suppository."
    2. "Get out of bed as soon as I get the suppository in place."
    3. "Try to hold the suppository for 15-20 minutes."
    4. "You will need to lay on your right side before I can insert this suppository."
22. How should the nurse administer rectal suppository medications? *(112)*
    1. They should be self-administered.
    2. Ask another nurse to give, as it is not pleasant to do.
    3. Discard the medication if a suppository becomes soft.
    4. Administer when the patient is lying on the left side.

23. List in order the procedure for administration of a disposable enema. *(113)*

    1. _____ Check pertinent patient monitoring parameters (i.e., last time defecated).
    2. _____ Explain carefully to the patient the procedure for administering an enema.
    3. _____ Put on gloves, remove protective covering from the rectal tube, and lubricate.
    4. _____ Position the patient on the left side and drape.
    5. _____ Remove and discard gloves and wash hands thoroughly.

24. When administering an enema to an adult, what does the nurse do? *(113)*

    1. Encourages the patient to hold the solution for about 5 minutes before defecating
    2. Heats the enema to 101° F to ensure comfort in administration
    3. Inserts 1 inch of the lubricated rectal tube into the rectum
    4. Tells the patient not to flush the toilet until the nurse returns and can see the results of the enema

Parenteral Administration: Safe Preparation of Parenteral Medications

chapter 9

Answer Key: Textbook page references are provided as a guide for answering these questions. A complete answer key is provided to your instructor.

MATCHING

Match the syringe on the right with the volume of medication on the left.

Volume of Medication

1. _____ tuberculin syringe
2. _____ 1-mL syringe
3. _____ 3-mL syringe
4. _____ 5-mL syringe
5. _____ 10-mL syringe

Syringe

a. 0.5 mL
b. 7.5 mL
c. 0.04 mL
d. 3.5 mL
e. 2 mL

REVIEW QUESTIONS

Identify the parts of a syringe and needle, as well as examples of the safety-type syringes and needles.

6. What is the outer portion of the syringe on which the calibrations for the measurements of drug volume are located called? *(117)*
   1. The gauge
   2. The barrel
   3. The tip
   4. The plunger
7. What is the inner cylindrical portion of the syringe that fits snugly into the barrel called? *(117)*
   1. The gauge
   2. The volume
   3. The tip
   4. The plunger
8. What is the portion of the syringe that holds the needle called? *(117)*
   1. The tip
   2. The gauge
   3. The barrel
   4. The plunger
9. The difference between a safety syringe and an ordinary syringe is that the safety syringe has which attachment? *(123)*
   1. The sleeve or sheath
   2. The needle cover
   3. The calibration measure
   4. The plunger topper

Describe how to select the correct needle gauge and length and how the needle gauge is determined.

10. The gauge of the needle is marked on the hub of the needle and on the outside of the disposable package; what does this number represent? *(119)*
    1. The length of the needle
    2. The inner diameter of the needle
    3. The actual dose the needle can hold
    4. The maximum volume allowed when using this needle
11. Which is an example of the gauge and length of a needle used for intradermal injection? *(121)*
    1. 25 gauge; 5/8 inch
    2. 18 gauge; 1 inch
    3. 29 gauge; 3/8 inch
    4. 20 gauge; 1/2 inch
12. The proper needle gauge is usually selected based on what factor? *(121)*
    1. The dose of the medication
    2. The site of injection
    3. The viscosity (thickness) of the solution
    4. The calibration scale used
13. Low-dose insulin syringes are used to measure insulin up to what dose? *(118)*
    1. 100 units
    2. 50 units
    3. 25 unit
    4. 10 units

14. What does the nurse instructing the patient on the use of an insulin pen include in the teaching? *(Select all that apply.)* **(119)**
    1. How to hold the pen correctly
    2. How to dial in the correct amount of insulin
    3. When to replace the cartridge
    4. How to refill the pen
    5. Which site to insert the needle and inject the proper dose

Compare and contrast the volumes of medications that can be measured in a tuberculin syringe and those of larger-volume syringes.

15. The nurse is preparing to give a subcutaneous injection of 0.5 mL of dalteparin. The medication should be injected using which syringe? **(119)**
    1. An insulin syringe
    2. A tuberculin syringe
    3. A prefilled syringe
    4. A standard plastic syringe
16. How is the use of the tuberculin syringe limited? **(117)**
    1. Only used for tuberculin inoculations
    2. Used for volumes smaller than 1 mL
    3. Only used for insulin administration
    4. Used for volumes greater than 1 mL
17. What are insulin syringes specifically calibrated to measure? **(118)**
    1. Doses of epinephrine
    2. Any volume smaller than 1 mL
    3. Volumes for tuberculin inoculations
    4. Doses of insulin only

Compare and contrast the advantages and disadvantages of using prefilled syringes.

18. The *advantages* of using a prefilled syringe include which factors? *(Select all that apply.)* **(119)**
    1. These syringes are to be used once and discarded.
    2. The time that is saved in preparing a standard amount of medication for one injection.
    3. The nurse can expect these syringes are cheaper than multi-vials.
    4. There is decreased chance for contamination using these syringes.
    5. A cartridge is required for use to hold the prefilled syringe.
19. The *disadvantages* of using a prefilled syringe include which factors? *(Select all that apply.)* **(119)**
    1. The nurse does not draw up the medication.
    2. An additional medication generally cannot be added to the cartridge.
    3. These syringes are to be used once and discarded.
    4. A cartridge is required for use to hold the prefilled syringe.
    5. The nurse can expect that these syringes are more expensive than multi-vials.

20. Many hospital pharmacies will use prefilled syringes for specific doses of medication for some patients, including what examples? *(Select all that apply.)* **(119)**
    1. Carpuject syringes
    2. Insulin pens
    3. Plastic syringes
    4. Tuberculin syringes
    5. EpiPen
21. The nurse was preparing to administer an intramuscular (IM) injection of 1 mg of Haldol, which was in a concentration of 1 mg/1 mL, to a confused patient. In the medication room, the nurse was choosing the correct needle and syringe from the shelf. The patient was an adult of normal weight, so the nurse selected which needle and syringe? **(121)**
    1. 25 gauge, 5/8-inch needle, with a 5-mL syringe
    2. 21 gauge, 1 1/2-inch needle, with a 3-mL syringe
    3. 29 gauge, 3/8-inch needle, with a 10-mL syringe
    4. 23 gauge, 1-inch needle, with an insulin syringe
22. Two nurses were in the medication room discussing the difference between the volume of medication that can be given in any subcutaneous site and the intradermal site. Which statement is correct? **(121)**
    1. "I always give between 0.5 mL and 1 mL for intradermal, and less than 0.1 mL for subcutaneous injections."
    2. "I always give between 0.01 mL and 0.1 mL for intradermal, and less than 1 mL for subcutaneous injections."
    3. "I always give between 0.01 mL and 0.1 mL for intradermal, and less than 2 mL for subcutaneous injections."
    4. "I always give between 0.1 mL and 1 mL for intradermal, and less than 0.5 mL for subcutaneous injections."
23. Which route is commonly thought to allow the medication to be absorbed rapidly? **(116)**
    1. Oral
    2. Rectal
    3. Intradermal
    4. Intramuscular

Differentiate among ampules, vials, and Mix-O-Vials.

24. What are glass containers that may be scored or have a darkened ring around the neck and usually contain a single dose of a medication called? **(126)**
    1. Ampules
    2. Metal lid vial
    3. Mix-O-Vials
    4. Rubber diaphragm vials
25. What are glass or plastic containers that contain one or more doses of a sterile medication called? **(126)**
    1. Vials
    2. Scored ampules
    3. Mix-O-Vials
    4. Ringed ampules

26. How does the nurse use a Mix-O-Vial? (A single dose of medication is normally contained in the Mix-O-Vial.) *(127)*
    1. By applying pressure to the rubber stopper between the two chambers
    2. By applying pressure to the top rubber diaphragm plunger
    3. By shaking the upper chamber (which contains the solvent) until it falls into the lower chamber (which contains the drug)
    4. By shaking the lower chamber (which contains the drug) until the upper chamber (which contains the solvent) falls down into the lower chamber

Describe the technique used to prepare two different drugs in one syringe (e.g., insulin).

27. When preparing NPH and Regular insulin together in the same syringe, what does the nurse need to do? *(127-129)*
    1. Discards NPH insulin if it is cloudy
    2. First draws up the NPH insulin to be administered
    3. First injects the amount of air equal to the amount of insulin to be withdrawn into the Regular insulin
    4. Is careful not to inject any of the first type of insulin already in the syringe into the vial

28. The nurse is preparing to administer 58 units of insulin and knows that which is true regarding insulin syringes? *(Select all that apply.)* *(118)*
    1. The shorter lines on the Regular insulin syringe represent 2 units measured.
    2. The longer lines on the low-dose insulin syringe measure 10 units of insulin.
    3. The low-dose insulin syringe can be used for this dose.
    4. The longer lines on the Regular insulin syringe measure 5 units of insulin.
    5. The shorter lines on the low-dose insulin syringe represent 1 unit measured.

29. List in order the correct sequence the nurse will follow to mix NPH and Regular insulin. *(127-129)*
    1. _____ Insert the needle into the NPH vial, and withdraw the correct amount of insulin.
    2. _____ Inject air into the Regular vial, invert the bottle, and withdraw the correct volume of Regular insulin.
    3. _____ Fill the syringe with air to an amount equal to the correct amount of NPH, insert the needle into the vial, inject air, remove needle.
    4. _____ Check the insulin prescription and wipe the tops of both vials of insulin.
    5. _____ Fill the syringe with air to an amount equal to the correct amount of Regular insulin.

Parenteral Administration: Intradermal, Subcutaneous, and Intramuscular Routes

Answer Key: Textbook page references are provided as a guide for answering these questions. A complete answer key is provided to your instructor.

MATCHING
Match the description on the right with the intramuscular site on the left.

Intramuscular Site

1. _____ vastus lateralis

2. _____ ventrogluteal

3. _____ rectus femoris

4. _____ deltoid

Description

a. Considered easiest site when patients are sitting
b. Considered easiest site for self-administration
c. Considered the preferred IM site for infants
d. Considered easiest site when patients are side-lying

REVIEW QUESTIONS

Describe the technique that is used to administer a medication via the intradermal route.

5. The most common site for the administration of intradermal medication is the inner aspect of which body part? *(133)*
   1. The shin
   2. The thigh
   3. The forearm
   4. The upper arm

6. When administering intradermal allergy testing for a patient, which steps does the nurse perform? *(Select all that apply.) (134-135)*
   1. Uses an alcohol wipe to clean the skin
   2. Wipes the site with alcohol after injection
   3. Aspirates for blood once the needle has been inserted
   4. Injects the volume ordered, usually 0.01-0.05 mL, into the subcutaneous tissue
   5. Asks the patient if any antihistamine or anti-inflammatory agents were taken 24-48 hours before the test

7. When preparing to provide allergy testing to a patient using the intradermal injection technique, what does the nurse do? *(134-135)*
   1. Performs hand hygiene and applies gloves
   2. Inserts the needle at a 90-degree angle with the needle bevel facing down
   3. Recaps the used needle before disposing of it in a puncture-resistant container
   4. Deposits the solution being injected into the subcutaneous tissue

List the equipment needed, and describe the technique that is used to administer a medication via the subcutaneous route.

8. The nurse is teaching a patient about the importance of rotating subcutaneous insulin injection sites. Which statement made by the patient indicates a need for additional teaching? *(136)*
   1. "The fastest site of absorption is when I inject into the abdomen."
   2. "Exercise will not affect the rate of insulin absorption."
   3. "Common subcutaneous sites for administering insulin include upper arms, anterior thighs, and the abdomen."
   4. "I need to rotate injection sites to prevent lipohypertrophy, which will slow insulin absorption."

9. Which route of injection is considered the fastest for medication absorption? *(135)*
   1. Intradermal
   2. Intraocular
   3. Subcutaneous
   4. Intramuscular

10. The nurse was educating a patient about heparin injections that would need to be continued at home, and the patient states, "I know that I need to inject my abdominal area just under the skin, right?" How should the nurse respond? *(135)*
    1. "That's correct, this is an intradermal injection."
    2. "Actually, this injection will go into the subcutaneous tissue, or the fat that is under the skin."
    3. "Well, this injection is designed to be delivered into your muscle, so instead of the abdomen, you will give it in your leg."
    4. "That is almost correct. It will go under your skin, but not in your abdomen; it will be in your arm."

Describe the technique used to administer medications intramuscularly.

11. The nurse is preparing to administer an IM injection in the ventrogluteal area. What does the nurse do first? *(139)*
    1. Positions the patient supine with the toes pointed outward
    2. Has the patient flex the gluteal muscle to minimize pain from the injection
    3. Identifies the site by forming a "V" on the lateral portion of the greater trochanter
    4. Holds the syringe at a 30-degree angle to the surface of the patient's skin

12. List the steps in order that the nurse will follow to administer an IM injection. *(140-141)*
    1. _____ Apply a small bandage to the site.
    2. _____ Explain carefully to the patient what will be done.
    3. _____ Insert the needle at the correct angle and depth for the site being used.
    4. _____ Carefully identify the patient using two patient identifiers.
    5. _____ Provide for privacy; position the patient appropriately.

13. What is the most important instruction to follow for the nurse administering an IM injection? *(140)*
    1. Add a bubble of air to the syringe.
    2. Pinch the skin into a bunch prior to injection.
    3. Tell the patient to hold his breath during the injection.
    4. Correctly identify the patient prior to administration.

Describe the landmarks that are used to identify the vastus lateralis muscle, the rectus femoris muscle, the ventrogluteal area, and the deltoid muscle before medication is administered.

14. When administering an IM injection in the deltoid muscle, the nurse will locate the site using which landmarks? *(139)*
    1. Finding the anterior lateral thigh
    2. Placing one hands-breadth below the greater trochanter
    3. Palpating the top of the shoulder and measuring down three finger-breadths
    4. From the crest of the ilium, directing the needle slightly upward

15. Which site for injection is located by placing the palm of the hand on the lateral portion of the greater trochanter, the thumb pointing toward the groin, the index finger on the anterior superior iliac spine, and the middle finger extended to the iliac crest? *(139)*
    1. The rectus femoris muscle
    2. The deltoid muscle
    3. The vastus lateralis muscle
    4. The ventrogluteal muscle

16. Where is the vastus lateralis muscle located? *(138)*
    1. In the buttock area
    2. On the thigh
    3. Below the shoulder
    4. Under the armpit

Identify suitable sites for the intramuscular administration of medication in an infant, a child, an adult, and an older adult.

17. Where is the best site for an IM injection for an infant? *(138)*
    1. The deltoid muscle
    2. The rectus femoris muscle
    3. The vastus lateralis muscle
    4. The ventrogluteal muscle

18. The nurse is planning to administer an IM injection for an adult patient who needs a flu vaccine (0.5 mL). Which muscle is the best to use? *(139)*
    1. The deltoid muscle
    2. The rectus femoris muscle
    3. The vastus lateralis muscle
    4. The ventrogluteal muscle

19. What does the nurse need to do before administering an IM injection into an older adult? *(Select all that apply.) (140-141)*
    1. Check the patient's allergy list.
    2. Verify the patient's identity using two identifiers.
    3. Cleanse the skin with an alcohol wipe.
    4. Ask another nurse to verify the correct dose prior to administration.
    5. Insert the needle to a depth of 1/2 inch and inject the medication.

Parenteral Administration: Intravenous Route

chapter

11

Answer Key: Textbook page references are provided as a guide for answering these questions. A complete answer key is provided to your instructor.

MATCHING
Match the definition on the right with the complication on the left.

Complication

1. _____ extravasation
2. _____ infiltration
3. _____ speed shock
4. _____ thrombophlebitis
5. _____ pulmonary edema
6. _____ septicemia
7. _____ localized infection
8. _____ phlebitis

Definition

a. symptoms include dyspnea, cough, coarse crackles, and frothy sputum
b. pathogens from a local infection invade the bloodstream causing fever and chills
c. an inflammation of a vein
d. the leakage of an intravenous solution into the surrounding tissue
e. redness, warmth, purulent drainage, swelling, and burning pain along the course of the vein
f. the leakage of an irritating chemical into the surrounding tissue
g. an inflammation of a vein with an associated blood clot
h. flushing, tightness in the chest, and hypotension

REVIEW QUESTIONS

Define intravenous (IV) therapy and describe the three intravascular compartments and the three fluid compartments of the body.

9. What are the three types of vessels that comprise the intravascular compartment? *(145)*
   1. The arterioles, alveoli, and veins
   2. The arteries, veins, and capillaries
   3. The sinuses, cavities, and pleural spaces
   4. The interstitial spaces, extracellular spaces, and intracellular spaces
10. What are the advantages of intravenous medications? *(Select all that apply.)* *(145)*
    1. This route is more comfortable than the subcutaneous route.
    2. The patient tends to be more mobile when using the intravenous route.
    3. Large volumes of fluids can be rapidly administered by this route.
    4. Medications can be directly injected into the vein using this route.
    5. The possibility of infection is decreased when using this route.

11. The spontaneous movement of water from an area of low electrolyte concentration to an area of high electrolyte concentration refers to a phenomenon that creates what? *(151)*
    1. Equilibrium
    2. Hydraulic pressure
    3. Osmotic pressure
    4. Electrolyte and protein compartments
12. What are the three fluid compartments of the body? *(145)*
    1. The arterioles, alveoli, and veins
    2. The arteries, veins, and capillaries
    3. The sinuses, cavities, and pleural spaces
    4. The interstitial spaces, intracellular spaces, and intravascular spaces
13. The fluid compartment that is composed of the intravascular and the interstitial compartment is known as what? *(145)*
    1. The intracellular compartment
    2. The extracellular compartment
    3. The intravenous compartment
    4. The extravenous compartment

Discuss the different IV access devices used for IV therapy.

14. What types of needles are used to access an implanted port? *(150)*
    1. Huber needles
    2. Subclavian needles
    3. Hickman needles
    4. Intravenous needles

15. What supplies does the nurse preparing to start an IV on a patient need? *(Select all that apply.) (158)*
    1. Sterile gloves
    2. Alcohol wipes
    3. Tourniquet
    4. Transparent dressing
    5. IV catheter

16. When calculating IV fluid rates, microdrip chambers form how many drops per milliliter? *(145)*
    1. 10
    2. 15
    3. 20
    4. 60

17. What are the common locations for peripheral IVs? *(Select all that apply.) (153)*
    1. The metacarpal veins
    2. The dorsal veins
    3. The jugular veins
    4. The basilic veins
    5. The cephalic veins

18. When a patient needs long-term IV or home IV therapy, the various types of catheters used will include which types? *(Select all that apply.) (149-150)*
    1. Peripherally inserted central catheters (PICC)
    2. Tunneled central venous catheters
    3. Implantable venous access devices
    4. Peripheral saline locks
    5. Hickman or Broviac catheters

19. Where are PICC lines inserted? *(149)*
    1. The jugular vein and threaded down to end at the superior vena cava
    2. The cephalic vein and threaded down to end at the superior vena cava
    3. The subclavian vein and threaded down to end at the superior vena cava
    4. The metacarpal vein and threaded down to end at the superior vena cava

Differentiate among isotonic, hypotonic, and hypertonic IV solutions and explain their clinical uses.

20. A patient has been admitted to the healthcare facility after experiencing a GI bleed at home, which has now resolved. The patient now has an intravascular fluid volume deficit. Which IV fluid does the nurse anticipate will be prescribed for the patient? *(151)*
    1. 0.9% sodium chloride
    2. 0.2% sodium chloride
    3. 0.45% sodium chloride
    4. 5% dextrose in water

21. Hypertonic solutions (e.g., parenteral nutrition solutions) are administered through central infusion lines directly into which blood vessel? *(152)*
    1. The inferior vena cava
    2. The jugular veins
    3. The peripheral veins
    4. The superior vena cava

22. Which type of solution contains fewer electrolytes and more free water? *(152)*
    1. Isotonic
    2. Hypotonic
    3. Hypertonic
    4. Replacement solutions

Identify the general principles for administering medications via the IV route.

23. Medications for IV administration are available in what dose forms? *(Select all that apply.) (152)*
    1. Vials
    2. Tablets
    3. Prefilled syringes
    4. Ampules
    5. Large-volume IV solution bags

24. In general, what does the nurse need to consider regarding any medication administered via the IV route? *(Select all that apply.) (154-155)*
    1. The SAS technique
    2. When an online filter is needed
    3. Use of appropriate barrier precautions
    4. Topical antibiotic creams are to be used on all insertion sites
    5. Used needles, syringes, and access devices are placed in puncture-resistant containers

25. Which types of catheters are used for IV administration? *(Select all that apply.) (148-149)*
    1. PICCs
    2. Midline catheters
    3. Peripheral venous catheters
    4. Central venous catheters
    5. Arterial catheters

Compare and contrast the differences between a peripheral IV line and a central IV line.

26. Which are examples of peripheral IV access devices? *(Select all that apply.) (148)*
    1. The butterfly needle
    2. The scalp needle
    3. The large-bore needle
    4. The winged needle
    5. The Huber needle

27. The nurse was teaching a patient about the need for a central IV access device and recognized further teaching was needed when the patient made which statement? *(149)*
    1. "I guess my veins in my arms are shot from the repeated IVs I have had, so a central line makes sense."
    2. "Since I will need to have long-term antibiotic therapy, it makes sense to have a PICC line."
    3. "I understand about Port-a-Caths since my wife's cousin had one for her chemotherapy."
    4. "As I understand it, this will mean that I will need to have my PICC changed every 3 months."

28. What are the advantages of a peripheral IV line over a central IV line? *(Select all that apply.)* *(148-149)*
    1. The peripheral line has fewer complications than the central line.
    2. The peripheral line is easier to insert than the central line.
    3. The peripheral line lasts longer than the central line.
    4. The peripheral line costs less than the central line.
    5. The peripheral line requires fewer assessments than the central line.

Describe the correct techniques for administering medications by means of a saline lock, an IV bag, an infusion pump, and a secondary piggyback set.

29. The nurse follows which steps when administering a medication by a saline lock? *(Select all that apply.)* *(160-161)*
    1. Selects a syringe several milliliters larger than that required by the volume of the drug.
    2. After determining that the IV has a blood return, injects saline for the flush followed by the medication at the rate specified by the manufacturer.
    3. After the medication is administered, inserts another syringe containing normal saline to flush the remaining drug from the catheter.
    4. Maintains constant pressure on the plunger of the syringe used to flush the line after the medication has been administered while simultaneously withdrawing the needle from the injection port to prevent backflow of blood.
    5. Verifies the saline dose with another qualified nurse.

30. The nurse is hanging a bag of normal saline for a patient who has been diagnosed with dehydration, and notices that the peripheral IV that was placed in the patient's hand has become dislodged. What should the nurse do next? *(172)*
    1. Advance the catheter into the vein.
    2. Resecure the catheter to the patient's hand.
    3. Remove the catheter and insert another one.
    4. Use the catheter, as it should migrate back into place.

31. While inserting an IV into a patient, the nurse has applied a tourniquet to help locate a vein. What other techniques are used in conjunction with a tourniquet to dilate the vein? *(Select all that apply.)* *(158)*
    1. Apply a heating pad.
    2. Apply cool, moist towels.
    3. Massage the vein.
    4. Place the extremity in a dependent position.
    5. Have the patient open and close his or her hand repeatedly.

Describe the recommended guidelines and procedures for IV catheter care.

32. Which statements about PICCs are correct? *(Select all that apply.)* *(149)*
    1. They are not available for pediatric use.
    2. PICC line insertion is only attempted in the operating room.
    3. PICCs cost less than other central venous catheters.
    4. PICC lines are easier to maintain than short peripheral catheters because the incidence of infiltration and phlebitis is less frequent.
    5. It is necessary to flush the PICC line with a saline-heparin solution after every use, or daily if not used.

33. When providing care to a patient receiving IV therapy, which actions does the nurse perform? *(Select all that apply.)* *(171-172)*
    1. Wears gloves to inspect the IV site
    2. Applies topical antibiotic ointment to the insertion site
    3. If it appears that the IV access device is clotted, attempts to clear the needle by flushing with fluid
    4. Checks the drip chamber; if it is less than half full, squeezes it to fill more completely
    5. Checks the temperature of the solution being infused because cold solutions can cause spasms in the vein

34. A patient has been ordered a PICC for the administration of medications. The nurse has taught the patient about the insertion procedure, use, and care of the PICC line. Which statement made by the patient indicates a need for further teaching? *(149)*
    1. "I will be able to go home with a PICC line."
    2. "My PICC line can last up to a year if it is properly cared for."
    3. "I will be placed under general anesthesia to have this intravenous line inserted."
    4. "The PICC line should be flushed with a saline-heparin solution after every use, or daily if not used."

Identify baseline assessments for IV therapy and proper maintenance of patency of IV lines and implanted access devices.

35. What are important teaching points to cover for patients and family members when discussing maintenance of central lines? *(168)*
    1. Patients need to be taught the signs and symptoms of infection.
    2. Patients need to be taught how to document the dressing change.
    3. Patients need to be taught how to reinsert the catheter when it accidently comes out.
    4. Patients need to be taught to carefully wrap any sharps in tissue paper and discard in the trash.

36. Which statements about implantable infusion ports are correct? *(Select all that apply.) (150)*
    1. Blood products can be administered through an implantable infusion port.
    2. One port of a two-port system may be reserved for drawing blood samples.
    3. An implanted central venous access catheter may remain in place for over a year and only requires a saline-heparin solution flush after every access or once monthly.
    4. The CDC recommends that central venous catheters be routinely replaced to prevent catheter-related infection.
    5. The infusion port can accommodate up to 100 punctures before it needs to be changed.

37. Important assessments for IV therapy are to determine when the IV needs to be: *(Select all that apply.) (149)*
    1. retaped and redressed.
    2. used for blood draws for labs.
    3. documented regarding the IV insertion site according to agency policy.
    4. flushed to determine the patency of the IV with fluids running.
    5. changed to another insertion site according to agency policy.

Explain the signs, symptoms, and treatment of the complications associated with IV therapy (e.g., phlebitis, thrombophlebitis, localized infection, septicemia, infiltration, extravasation, air in tubing, pulmonary edema, catheter embolism, and "speed shock").

38. The nurse will monitor the patient with an IV for signs and symptoms of the inflammation of a vein, which is called: *(172)*
    1. extravasation.
    2. thrombus.
    3. phlebitis.
    4. thrombophlebitis.

39. What are the implications of the complication of extravasation in patients with IV drug drips and medications given IV push? *(173)*
    1. Serious tissue damage may occur.
    2. The needle tip has punctured the vein.
    3. The patient is now becoming infected.
    4. The patient will experience warmth, tenderness, swelling, and burning pain in the IV site.

40. The nurse recognizes circulatory overload in a patient experiencing which symptoms while receiving IV therapy? *(174)*
    1. Dyspnea, hypertension, anxiety, and fever
    2. Dyspnea, pleuritic pain, sweating, tachycardia, cough, and cyanosis
    3. Dyspnea, cough, anxiety, rhonchi, and possible cardiac dysrhythmias
    4. Engorged neck veins, dyspnea, reduced urine output, edema, bounding pulse, and shallow rapid respirations

Drugs That Affect the Autonomic Nervous System

chapter
12

Answer Key: Textbook page references are provided as a guide for answering these questions. A complete answer key is provided to your instructor.

MATCHING
Match the sympathetic or parasympathetic nervous system on the right with the action on the left. Insert "a" for sympathetic or "b" for parasympathetic.

Actions

1. _____ relaxation of the GI sphincters
2. _____ dilation of the pupil in the eye (mydriasis)
3. _____ relaxation of the bronchial muscles
4. _____ constriction of the systemic veins
5. _____ constriction of the bronchial muscles
6. _____ constriction of the pupil in the eye (miosis)
7. _____ constriction of the GI sphincters
8. _____ relaxation of the bladder sphincter (urinary)

Sympathetic or Parasympathetic Nervous System

a. sympathetic or adrenergic receptors
b. parasympathetic or cholinergic receptors

REVIEW QUESTIONS

Scenario: A 69-year-old male was admitted to the hospital with an exacerbation of his asthma. He has a history of hypertension, diabetes, and benign prostatic hyperplasia (BPH).

Describe how the central nervous system differs from the peripheral nervous system.

9. What is the primary difference between the central nervous system (CNS) and the peripheral nervous system (PNS)? *(177)*
   1. CNS controls the autonomic nervous system, while the PNS controls the motor nervous system.
   2. CNS is comprised of afferent and efferent nerves, while the PNS is comprised of the brain and the spinal cord.
   3. CNS controls all involuntary movements and the PNS controls all voluntary movements.
   4. CNS is comprised of the brain and the spinal cord, while the PNS is comprised of afferent and efferent nerves.

10. The PNS is further subdivided into the somatic nervous system that controls voluntary movement and which other system? *(177)*
    1. The vascular system
    2. The endocrine system
    3. The autonomic nervous system
    4. The system of neurotransmitters
11. What primary function is controlled by the somatic nervous system? *(177)*
    1. Skeletal muscle contractions
    2. Secretion of enzymes into the digestive system
    3. Involuntary contraction of the digestive system
    4. Transmission of neuronal impulses within the synaptic junctions
12. Once a neurotransmitter has been released into the synaptic junction, what happens then? *(178)*
    1. A receptor is activated on the next neuron in the chain.
    2. A decrease in response to nerve stimulation occurs.
    3. The neurotransmitter activates the fight-or-flight response.
    4. Symptoms of Parkinson's disease become apparent.

13. Neurotransmitters that are released into synapses at the end of neurons are able to cause which reaction? *(Select all that apply.)* **(178)**
    1. Secrete an enzyme.
    2. Release a second neurotransmitter.
    3. Stimulate receptors on an end organ.
    4. Inhibit electrical impulses through the neuron.
    5. Respond by secreting another neurotransmitter.
14. What are examples of end-organ receptors that are part of the nervous system and are usually at the end of the nerve chain? *(Select all that apply.)* **(178)**
    1. The brain
    2. The spinal cord
    3. The adrenal glands
    4. The heart muscle
    5. The smooth muscles of the GI tract

Name the most common neurotransmitters known to affect central nervous system function and identify the two major neurotransmitters of the autonomic nervous system.

15. What are the major types of receptors found in the autonomic nervous system? *(Select all that apply.)* **(178)**
    1. Alpha
    2. Beta
    3. Dopaminergic
    4. Gamma
    5. Delta
16. What are the nerve endings that liberate acetylcholine? **(178)**
    1. The adrenergic fibers
    2. The cholinergic fibers
    3. The cholinergic agents
    4. The adrenergic agents
17. What are the two major neurotransmitters of the autonomic nervous system? **(178)**
    1. Norepinephrine and acetylcholine
    2. Epinephrine and acetylcholine
    3. Epinephrine and dopamine
    4. Norepinephrine and epinephrine
18. Which system controls blood pressure and body temperature? **(178)**
    1. Motor nervous system
    2. Voluntary nervous system
    3. Autonomic nervous system
    4. Somatic nervous system

Explain how drugs inhibit the actions of cholinergic and adrenergic fibers.

19. Which medications cause effects similar to those produced by the adrenergic neurotransmitter norepinephrine? **(178)**
    1. Adrenergic agents
    2. Cholinergic agents
    3. Anticholinergic agents
    4. Adrenergic-blocking agents

20. Which are medications used to inhibit the effects of the natural neurotransmitter acetylcholine secreted by cholinergic fibers? **(178)**
    1. Adrenergic agents
    2. Cholinergic agents
    3. Anticholinergic agents
    4. Adrenergic-blocking agents
21. Which are medications used to inhibit the effects of the natural catecholamines secreted by the adrenergic fibers? **(178)**
    1. Adrenergic agents
    2. Cholinergic agents
    3. Anticholinergic agents
    4. Adrenergic-blocking agents
22. Cholinergic fibers are those nerve endings that secrete which neurotransmitter? **(178)**
    1. Histamine
    2. Acetylcholine
    3. Dopamine
    4. Norepinephrine

Identify two broad classes of drugs used to stimulate the adrenergic nervous system.

23. Since the cholinergic agents and the adrenergic agents have opposite effects, the medications that slow down heart rates and cause pupillary constriction (miosis) are which type of agents? **(179)**
    1. Cholinergic agents
    2. Adrenergic-blocking agents
    3. Anticholinergic agents
    4. Adrenergic agents
24. Which class of drugs has the opposite effect of the cholinergic agents and causes pupillary dilation (mydriasis) and rapid heart rate? **(178)**
    1. Cholinergic agents
    2. Adrenergic-blocking agents
    3. Anticholinergic agents
    4. Adrenergic agents
25. Adrenergic fibers are nerve endings that secrete which neurotransmitter? **(178)**
    1. Histamine
    2. Acetylcholine
    3. Dopamine
    4. Norepinephrine
26. Which are catecholamines produced primarily from nerve terminals; the adrenal medulla; and selected sites in the brain, kidneys, and GI tract? **(178)**
    1. Enkephalins, endorphins, and histamine
    2. Dopamine, glycine, and gamma-aminobutyric acid
    3. Norepinephrine, epinephrine, and dopamine
    4. Prostaglandins, histamine, and cyclic adenosine monophosphate (cAMP)

27. Which catecholamines are secreted naturally in the body? *(Select all that apply.)* *(178)*
    1. Dopamine
    2. Acetylcholine
    3. Epinephrine
    4. Serotonin
    5. Norepinephrine

Review the actions of adrenergic agents and the conditions that require the use of these drugs.

28. A nurse was reviewing the prescription for albuterol (Proventil, Ventolin), an adrenergic agent used for the patient in the scenario, and remembered that this agent can cause which effect in patients with diabetes? *(179)*
    1. Hypotension
    2. Allergic reactions
    3. Hyperglycemia
    4. Hypoglycemia

29. The patient in the scenario experiences orthostatic hypotension as a result of taking a beta-adrenergic blocking agent for treatment of hypertension. Which measures does the nurse incorporate into this patient's plan of care? *(Select all that apply.)* *(180)*
    1. Discontinue the beta-adrenergic-blocking agent.
    2. Instruct the patient to avoid standing for long periods.
    3. Encourage the patient to sit down if feeling faint.
    4. Teach the patient to rise slowly from a supine or sitting position.
    5. Teach the patient to perform exercises to prevent blood pooling in the extremities when standing or sitting for long periods.

30. Stimulation of the adrenergic receptors causes the smooth muscle of the bronchial tree to relax, which results in what effect? *(179)*
    1. Stridor
    2. Wheezing
    3. Bronchodilation
    4. Bronchoconstriction

Describe the benefits of using beta-adrenergic blocking agents for hypertension, angina pectoris, cardiac dysrhythmias, and hyperthyroidism.

31. Stimulation of beta$_2$ receptors in a patient results in which assessment findings? *(Select all that apply.)* *(182)*
    1. Bronchoconstriction
    2. Uterine relaxation
    3. Bronchodilation
    4. Pupil constriction (miosis)
    5. Vasodilation of peripheral blood vessels

32. Which medication is the preferred treatment for the patient in the scenario with asthma in need of treatment with a beta blocker? *(182)*
    1. Propranolol
    2. Timolol
    3. Nadolol
    4. Atenolol

33. What are serious adverse effects of beta-adrenergic blocking agent therapy? *(Select all that apply.)* *(184)*
    1. Nausea
    2. Bradycardia
    3. Wheezing
    4. Orthopnea
    5. Headache

Identify diseases in which beta-adrenergic blocking agents should not be used, and discuss why they should not be used.

34. Beta-adrenergic blocking agents such as carvedilol (Coreg) must be used with caution in diabetic patients because these agents may induce, as well as mask, the signs of what? *(182)*
    1. Wheezing
    2. Tachycardia
    3. Hypoglycemia
    4. Hyperglycemia

35. What is a possible effect of administering beta blockers to the patient in the scenario with a known respiratory disease such as asthma? *(182)*
    1. Hyperglycemia
    2. Hypertension
    3. Bronchodilation
    4. Bronchoconstriction

36. Since beta-adrenergic blocking agents have the potential to cause hypotension, bradycardia, and heart failure, it is important to monitor for an increase in which symptoms of heart failure? *(Select all that apply.)* *(184)*
    1. Edema
    2. Crackles
    3. Dyspnea
    4. Urinary retention
    5. Hypoglycemia

Describe clinical uses and the predictable adverse effects of cholinergic agents and anticholinergic agents.

37. Patients with which condition would most likely benefit from the dopaminergic effects of adrenergic agents? *(178)*
    1. Parkinson's disease
    2. Guillain-Barré syndrome
    3. Amyotrophic lateral sclerosis
    4. Multiple sclerosis

38. For patients who have benign prostatic hyperplasia and difficulty voiding, which class of drugs help by increasing contractions of the urinary bladder? *(184)*
    1. Anticholinergic agents
    2. Adrenergic agents
    3. Cholinergic agents
    4. Adrenergic-blocking agents

39. Anticholinergic agents are used clinically in the treatment of which disorders? *(Select all that apply.)* *(185)*
    1. Glaucoma
    2. Infant colic
    3. Urinary retention
    4. Irritable bowel syndrome
    5. Reducing bronchial secretions presurgery

Drugs Used for Sleep

Answer Key: Textbook page references are provided as a guide for answering these questions. A complete answer key is provided to your instructor.

MATCHING

Match the definition on the right with the sleep patterns on the left.

Sleep Pattern

1. _____ insomnia
2. _____ initial insomnia
3. _____ intermittent insomnia
4. _____ terminal insomnia
5. _____ short-term insomnia
6. _____ chronic insomnia
7. _____ rebound sleep

Definition

a. at least 1 month of sleep disturbance
b. the inability to fall asleep when desired
c. early awakening with the inability to fall asleep again
d. compensatory REM sleep
e. the inability to sleep
f. a sleep disturbance that lasts less than 3 weeks,
g. the inability to stay asleep

REVIEW QUESTIONS

Scenario: A nurse was taking care of a 58-year-old patient who complained of not being able to sleep. To understand the exact problem, the nurse asked the patient if she was having trouble getting to sleep or if she woke up during the night and could not get back to sleep.

Differentiate among the terms *sedative* and *hypnotic; initial, intermittent,* and *terminal insomnia;* and *short-term* and *chronic insomnia* and *rebound sleep.*

8. The nurse's questions to the patient in the scenario are intended to determine if there is which type of insomnia? *(189)*
   1. Initial insomnia or rebound insomnia
   2. Initial insomnia or intermittent insomnia
   3. Initial insomnia or terminal insomnia
   4. Initial insomnia or transient insomnia
9. The nurse knows which classification of drugs can be used for patients complaining of insomnia? *(Select all that apply.) (189)*
   1. Hypnotics
   2. Sedatives
   3. Antidepressants
   4. Anticonvulsants
   5. Anticholinergics

10. The phrase *rebound sleep* refers to what phenomenon? *(189)*
    1. The return to previous insomnia symptoms
    2. The increase in amount of REM sleep that causes restlessness and vivid nightmares
    3. The return of normal sleep patterns after a hypnotic is discontinued
    4. The decrease in the amount of REM sleep that causes increased drowsiness
11. After discussing with the patient in the scenario the best drugs to use for insomnia, the nurse recognizes the need for further education when the patient makes which statement? *(189)*
    1. "So you are saying that I should take drugs for my insomnia for short periods of time to prevent the side effects."
    2. "I see; if I use a hypnotic prior to going to bed this will help with my insomnia."
    3. "You are right. If I don't start getting better sleep it will start to interfere with my work."
    4. "So you are saying that the best type of drug to use for insomnia is a sedative."

12. How is *insomnia* best defined? *(189)*
    1. The inability to sleep
    2. Getting fewer than 5 hours of sleep a night
    3. Episodes of REM sleep that last only a few minutes
    4. Experiencing a drifting or floating sensation

Identify alterations found in the sleep pattern when hypnotics are discontinued.

13. The nurse teaching a patient about the use of hypnotics and what to expect when they are discontinued recognized the need for further instruction when the patient made which statement? *(189)*
    1. "As I understand it, sedatives have the same effect as hypnotic medications."
    2. "Habitual use of benzodiazepines may result in physical dependence."
    3. "Since some of these drugs have unpleasant consequences such as rebound sleep, I will need to change my habits instead of relying on medications to sleep."
    4. "Insomnia is not a disease, but a symptom of the stress I am having since I became unemployed."

14. Which medications and/or substances does the nurse identify as potentially inducing or aggravating insomnia? *(Select all that apply.)* *(190)*
    1. Alcohol
    2. Caffeine
    3. Nicotine
    4. Benzodiazepines
    5. Anticonvulsants

15. After long-term administration of sedative-hypnotic agents, the patient may experience what if the medications are discontinued? *(Select all that apply.)* *(189)*
    1. Drowsiness
    2. Restlessness
    3. Vivid nightmares
    4. Severe REM rebound sleep
    5. Quick return of normal sleep patterns

Cite nursing interventions that can be implemented as an alternative to administering a sedative-hypnotic medication.

16. While teaching patients about nonpharmacologic methods to enhance sleep, which statement does the nurse include? *(190)*
    1. "Exercise during the day, not near bedtime."
    2. "Avoid drinking milk before going to bed."
    3. "Do not go to bed at the same time each night; go to bed when you feel the most tired."
    4. "Eat your heaviest meal of the day about 45 minutes before you plan to go to bed."

17. The nurse knows that the patient who has complained of insomnia can benefit from which alternative methods of inducing sleep? *(Select all that apply.)* *(190)*
    1. A limitation of stimulants close to bedtime
    2. Avoiding heavy meals late in the evening
    3. Drinking warm milk and eating crackers as a bedtime snack
    4. Limiting exercise during the day and only within 30 minutes of bedtime
    5. Consuming only decaffeinated beverages close to bedtime

18. The nurse was reviewing a diet choice made by a patient who was suffering from insomnia. Which choice would be a good alternative to a sedative? *(190)*
    1. Chocolate bar and hot milk
    2. Herbal tea and crackers
    3. Hot black tea and a cookie before bed
    4. Glass of wine and dark chocolate

Compare the effects of benzodiazepines and nonbenzodiazepines on the central nervous system.

19. Which statements does the nurse include when teaching a patient about zolpidem (Ambien) therapy? *(194)*
    1. "No physical dependency will develop with use of this drug."
    2. "If you have difficulty sleeping, increase the dose by one-half."
    3. "Take the medication about 3 hours before you plan on going to sleep."
    4. "The 'morning hangover' side effect is generally not a problem with this medication."

20. How does the drug class benzodiazepines work? *(191)*
    1. By activating the sleep function of the cerebral cortex
    2. By suppressing REM and stages III and IV sleep patterns
    3. By stimulating the neurotransmitter dopamine that initiates sleep
    4. By binding to receptors that stimulate the release of gamma-aminobutyric acid (GABA)

21. The drug class nonbenzodiazepines, which include the benzodiazepine receptor agonists (e.g., zaleplon, zolpidem, eszopiclone), have which adverse effect that requires careful monitoring? *(196-197)*
    1. Food slows the absorption of the drug.
    2. Lightheadedness lasts for several moments and passes.
    3. Habitual use may result in physical dependence.
    4. An ultra–short-acting time that affects the tolerance to the drug.

Identify the antidote drug used for the management of benzodiazepine overdose.

22. What do the therapeutic outcomes of benzodiazepine therapy include? *(Select all that apply.)* **(192)**
    1. To produce mild sedation
    2. To use short-term to produce sleep
    3. To manage migraine headaches
    4. To induce preoperative sedation with amnesia
    5. To increase the amount of REM sleep

23. A nurse was caring for a 54-year-old patient who was admitted for benzodiazepine overdose after taking over 20 lorazepam (Ativan) tablets. The nurse expects which medication to be prescribed for the treatment of the overdose? **(192)**
    1. quazepam (Doral)
    2. flumazenil (Romazicon)
    3. triazolam (Halcion)
    4. eszopiclone (Lunesta)

24. Rapid discontinuance of benzodiazepines after long-term use may result in symptoms similar to those of alcohol withdrawal, which include: *(Select all that apply.)* **(192)**
    1. delirium.
    2. headaches.
    3. weakness.
    4. anxiety.
    5. grand mal seizures.

Identify laboratory tests that should be monitored when benzodiazepines are administered for an extended period.

25. Since one of the common adverse effects of benzodiazepines is blood dyscrasias, the nurse will monitor which lab values? *(Select all that apply.)* **(194)**
    1. Platelets
    2. Red blood cells
    3. Electrolytes
    4. Prothrombin time
    5. White blood cells with differential

26. The symptoms of hepatotoxicity are anorexia, nausea, vomiting, jaundice, hepatomegaly, splenomegaly, and abnormal liver function tests, which include what results? *(Select all that apply.)* **(194)**
    1. Bilirubin
    2. Platelets
    3. Alkaline phosphatase
    4. Aspartate aminotransferase [AST]
    5. Alanine aminotransferase [ALT]

27. Why may a pregnancy test be ordered when a patient is started on a benzodiazepine? **(192)**
    1. These agents cross into breast milk.
    2. The withdrawal symptoms are worse for pregnant mothers.
    3. There is an increased incidence of maternal deaths after use of these drugs.
    4. There is an increased incidence of birth defects because these agents cross the placenta.

Drugs Used to Treat Neurodegenerative Disorders

Answer Key: Textbook page references are provided as a guide for answering these questions. A complete answer key is provided to your instructor.

MATCHING

Match the definition to the terminology used in neurodegenerative disorders.

Definition

1. _____ a lack of movement

2. _____ quick, short steps that may be forward or backward unintentionally

3. _____ a diffuse rose-colored mottling of the skin

4. _____ a chronic, progressive disorder of the central nervous system causing movement disorders

5. _____ a progressive neurodegenerative disease causing cognitive dysfunction

6. _____ a shaking often observed in the hands, and may involve the jaws, lips, and tongue

7. _____ an impairment of the ability to perform voluntary movement

Neurodegenerative terminology

a. Parkinson's disease
b. Alzheimer's disease
c. dyskinesia
d. akinesia
e. tremors
f. livedo reticularis
g. propulsive, uncontrolled movement

REVIEW QUESTIONS

Scenario: A 57-year-old patient who was diagnosed with Parkinson's disease is admitted to an inpatient unit to regulate his medications.

Identify the signs and symptoms of Parkinson's disease.

8. The nurse caring for the patient in the scenario expects to see the patient exhibit symptoms that include difficulty walking and possibly stooped posture, as well as what other symptoms? *(Select all that apply.)* **(200)**
   1. Muscle tremors
   2. Urinary retention
   3. Muscle weakness with rigidity
   4. Posture and equilibrium changes
   5. Slowness of movement in performing daily activities

9. Parkinson's disease is caused by a deterioration of what? **(199)**
   1. The levodopa receptors
   2. The dopaminergic neurons
   3. The cholinergic fibers
   4. The acetylcholine neurons

10. Although Parkinson's disease is primarily considered a disease that affects the patient's ability to walk, it also has nonmotor symptoms such as what? *(Select all that apply.)* **(200)**
    1. Orthostatic hypotension
    2. Nocturnal sleep disturbances
    3. Nausea and vomiting
    4. Daytime somnolence
    5. Bladder incontinence

11. Which classification of drugs is used to treat parkinsonism by reducing the metabolism of dopamine in the brain? **(210)**
    1. COMT inhibitors
    2. Anticholinergic agents
    3. Monoamine oxidase type B inhibitors
    4. Selective serotonin reuptake inhibitors

12. Which agents are used in the treatment of Parkinson's disease primarily because they provide symptomatic relief from excessive acetylcholine? *(201)*
    1. Dopamine agonists
    2. Anticholinergic agents
    3. Monoamine oxidase type B inhibitors
    4. Selective serotonin reuptake inhibitors
13. Which symptom of Parkinson's disease is manifested as extremely slow body movements that may eventually progress to a total lack of movement? *(203)*
    1. Akinesia
    2. Dyskinesia
    3. Bradykinesia
    4. Propulsive movement

Identify the neurotransmitter that is found in excess and the neurotransmitter that is deficient in people with parkinsonism.

14. With Parkinson's disease, which neurotransmitter is deficient? *(199)*
    1. Norepinephrine
    2. Dopamine
    3. Serotonin
    4. Acetylcholine
15. What is the neurotransmitter that is considered to be in excess in Parkinson's disease? *(199)*
    1. Serotonin
    2. Norepinephrine
    3. Acetylcholine
    4. Dopamine
16. What can be a cause of secondary parkinsonism? *(Select all that apply.)* *(200)*
    1. Tumors
    2. Hereditary
    3. Intracranial infections
    4. Head trauma
    5. Unknown causes

Describe the reasonable expectations of the medications that are prescribed for the treatment of Parkinson's disease.

17. What is the goal of treatment for Parkinson's disease? *(Select all that apply.)* *(201)*
    1. Cure the disease.
    2. Moderate the symptoms of the disease.
    3. Slow the progression of the disease.
    4. Speed up the absorption of dopamine.
    5. Slow the deterioration of acetylcholine.
18. Which statement does the nurse include when teaching a patient with Parkinson's disease about the drug apomorphine (Apokyn)? *(209)*
    1. It is administered intravenously.
    2. It is chemically related to morphine, but does not have any opioid activity.
    3. It is used to treat hypermobility associated with the "weaning off" of dopamine agonists.
    4. It commonly causes hypertension in patients who initially start therapy with this drug.

19. Which medication used in treating patients with Parkinson's disease reduces the destruction of dopamine in the peripheral tissues, allowing significantly more dopamine to reach the brain to eliminate the symptoms of parkinsonism? *(214)*
    1. entacapone (Comtan)
    2. ropinirole (Requip)
    3. apomorphine (Apokyn)
    4. selegiline (Eldepryl)
20. Generally, patients with Parkinson's disease will be treated with carbidopa-levodopa, but the drug's effect gradually wears off by which time? *(206)*
    1. In 12-24 months
    2. In 3-5 years
    3. In 1-2 years
    4. In 6-8 months
21. When patients start on monoamine oxidase type B inhibitor therapy in conjunction with carbidopa-levodopa (Sinemet), the dosages of Sinemet can be titrated downward starting when? *(205)*
    1. After month 4 or 5 of therapy
    2. After month 2 or 3 of therapy
    3. After week 2 or 3 of therapy
    4. After day 2 or 3 of therapy
22. What is the term for when the drugs used for Parkinson's disease start to become ineffective? *(204)*
    1. Hypermobility
    2. Neuroprotective
    3. A common adverse effect
    4. The on-off phenomenon

Cite the action of carbidopa, levodopa, and apomorphine on the neurotransmitters involved in Parkinson's disease.

23. What is the major action of the drug carbidopa when combined with levodopa? *(206)*
    1. To reduce dopamine production
    2. To reduce metabolism of levodopa
    3. To increase the metabolism of levodopa
    4. To absorb more levodopa
24. The drugs carbidopa-levodopa (Sinemet) must be given in combination because of which effect? *(206)*
    1. Levodopa has no effect when used alone.
    2. Carbidopa has no effect when used alone.
    3. Levodopa is used to reduce the dose of carbidopa required.
    4. Carbidopa is used to increase the dose of levodopa required.

25. Which are nursing considerations for patients on apomorphine (Apokyn) therapy? *(Select all that apply.)* *(209-210)*
    1. Do not administer apomorphine intravenously.
    2. Calculate apomorphine dose based on milligrams.
    3. Administer prochlorperazine for nausea associated with apomorphine therapy.
    4. Assess patients on apomorphine therapy for orthostatic hypotension.
    5. Assess patients receiving apomorphine therapy for sudden sleep attacks.

Explain the action of entacapone and of the monoamine oxidase inhibitors (selegiline and rasagiline) as it relates to the treatment of Parkinson's disease.

26. What is the major action of the drug entacapone (Comtan), which is a COMT inhibitor? *(214)*
    1. Increase the absorption of dopamine.
    2. Slow the progression of deterioration of dopaminergic nerve cells.
    3. Increase the adverse dopaminergic effects of levodopa.
    4. Reduce the destruction of dopamine in the peripheral tissues.
27. Active metabolites of selegiline (Eldepryl), when swallowed, are amphetamines that cause cardiovascular and psychiatric adverse effects. To avoid this effect, how is the drug administered? *(204)*
    1. A rectal suppository
    2. A subcutaneous injection
    3. An orally disintegrating tablet
    4. An intradermal injection

Cite the specific symptoms that should show improvement when anticholinergic agents are administered to a patient with Parkinson's disease.

28. What are the therapeutic outcomes expected for a patient after being treated for Parkinson's disease with anticholinergic agents? *(Select all that apply.)* *(216)*
    1. Improvement in their gait and posture
    2. Decreased depression level and improved mood
    3. Improvement in speech pattern
    4. Decrease in drooling
    5. Decrease in the severity of the tremors
29. What is the main reason anticholinergic agents are prescribed for patients with parkinsonism? *(216)*
    1. Decrease the absorption of acetylcholine
    2. Increase the absorption of dopamine
    3. Reduce hyperstimulation caused by the excess amount of acetylcholine
    4. Prevent the adverse effect of orthostatic hypotension

30. What nursing assessments are needed for patients who are starting on carbidopa-levodopa therapy? *(206)*
    1. Perform a baseline assessment using UPDRS.
    2. Plan to perform a baseline assessment every 3 months while on the drug.
    3. Observe for the drug's therapeutic effect to occur within 2 weeks of therapy.
    4. Anticipate the patient developing livedo reticularis within 2 weeks of therapy.
31. Anticholinergic agents produce which effects? *(Select all that apply.)* *(216-217)*
    1. Dry mouth
    2. Diarrhea
    3. Runny nose
    4. Dry nose
    5. Constipation

Explain the action of the agents used in the treatment of Alzheimer's disease.

32. What is the primary action of donepezil (Aricept)? *(218)*
    1. It prevents the loss of cholinergic neurons.
    2. It allows norepinephrine to accumulate at the neuron synapses.
    3. It inhibits acetylcholinesterase, the enzyme that breaks down acetylcholine.
    4. It activates acetylcholinesterase, the enzyme that breaks down acetylcholine.
33. What is the primary therapeutic outcome of memantine (Namenda)? *(219)*
    1. The enhancement of muscle tone
    2. The improvement of cognitive skills
    3. The improvement of mobility and coordination
    4. The prevention or slowing of the neurodegeneration of Alzheimer's disease
34. Which statements does the nurse include when teaching a patient and family about donepezil (Aricept)? *(Select all that apply.)* *(219)*
    1. "Donepezil must be taken on an empty stomach."
    2. "This drug will prevent your disease from getting worse."
    3. "Notify your healthcare provider if your pulse is fewer than 60 beats per minute."
    4. "Discontinue the drug if you develop diarrhea early in the treatment program."
    5. "You may feel a little nauseated when first taking this medication, but this usually subsides after 2-3 weeks of therapy."

Drugs Used for Anxiety Disorders

Answer Key: Textbook page references are provided as a guide for answering these questions. A complete answer key is provided to your instructor.

MATCHING

Match the definition on the right with the term on the left.

Term

1. _____ anxiety
2. _____ panic
3. _____ phobias
4. _____ obsessive-compulsive

Definition

a. an abrupt surge of intense fear or intense discomfort
b. excessive and unrealistic worry about two or more life circumstances
c. recurrent thoughts or actions that cause significant distress and interfere with normal functioning
d. irrational fears of specific objects, activities, or situations

REVIEW QUESTIONS

Scenario: A 58-year-old patient was admitted for further evaluation of bizarre behavior manifested as loud, rapid talking; pacing; and wringing of the hands. Relatives have attempted to calm the patient with no effect, and they brought the patient to urgent care for consultation.

Compare and contrast the differences among generalized anxiety disorder, panic disorder, phobias, and obsessive-compulsive disorder.

5. When patients have irrational fears of a specific object, activity, or situation, and even recognize the fear as exaggerated or unrealistic, this is termed what? *(223)*
   1. A phobia
   2. A panic disorder
   3. An allergic response
   4. An obsessive-compulsive disorder
6. Patients may which have physiological symptoms of anxiety? *(Select all that apply.)* *(222)*
   1. Tachycardia
   2. Muscle spasms
   3. Palpitations
   4. Increased urination
   5. Sweating
7. When patients have unwanted thoughts, ideas, images, or an urge that the patient recognizes as time-consuming and senseless but repeatedly intrudes into the consciousness despite attempts to ignore,

prevent, or counteract it, the patient is said to be experiencing what? *(223)*
   1. A phobia
   2. A panic disorder
   3. An allergic response
   4. An obsessive-compulsive disorder

Describe the essential components included in a baseline assessment of a patient's mental status.

8. In the scenario, the nurse will regularly assess the patient for which symptoms to determine if acute hospitalization is indicated? *(224)*
   1. Patient is complaining of nausea and refuses breakfast.
   2. Patient appears to be at risk for harming him- or herself or others.
   3. Patient has a clean and neat appearance, and the ability to perform self-care.
   4. Patient demonstrates a stooped or slumped posture, and is oriented to date, time, place, and person.
9. Why is it important for the nurse to identify events that trigger anxiety? *(225)*
   1. To be aware of what to avoid talking about with the patient
   2. To reintroduce the trigger in a controlled environment and cure the patient of their anxiety
   3. To question the validity of the anxiety to help the patient see how foolish it is
   4. To help the patient to reduce anxiety or cope more adaptively with stressors

10. The nurse is taking care of the patient in the scenario and performs a baseline mental status assessment, which will include asking the patient to describe what normal patterns? *(Select all that apply.)* **(224)**
    1. Sleep
    2. Weight gains or losses
    3. Family interactions
    4. Psychomotor functions
    5. Obsessions or compulsions

Cite the drug therapy used to treat anxiety disorders.

11. Which drug classes are used to treat patients with anxiety disorders? *(Select all that apply.)* **(227)**
    1. Benzodiazepines
    2. Azaspirones
    3. Calcium channel blockers
    4. Selective serotonin reuptake inhibitors (SSRIs)
    5. Monoamine oxidase type B inhibitors

12. Hydroxyzine therapy is used for patients who suffer from conditions characterized by anxiety, tension, and agitation, because it has which effect? **(229)**
    1. Antihistaminic
    2. Antiemetic
    3. Antianxiety
    4. Antispasmodic

13. The nursing implications for buspirone therapy include watching for symptoms of which adverse effects of the drug? *(Select all that apply.)* **(228)**
    1. Dizziness and insomnia
    2. Orthostatic hypotension
    3. Sedation and lethargy
    4. Nervousness and drowsiness
    5. Restless leg syndrome

14. The benzodiazepine drug monograph lists hepatotoxicity as a serious adverse effect. Which laboratory tests are performed to assess this? **(228)**
    1. Creatinine, creatinine clearance, and albumin
    2. Albumin, ferritin, and prothrombin time
    3. Aspartate aminotransferase (AST), alanine aminotransferase (ALT), and alkaline phosphatase
    4. Hemoglobin, alkaline phosphatase, and prothrombin time

Identify adverse effects that may result from drug therapy used to treat anxiety.

15. When determining if drug therapy is effective for patients taking fluvoxamine (Luvox) as an antianxiety agent, the nurse will note which characteristics of the patient's behavior? **(229)**
    1. Slurred speech and dizziness occur.
    2. Coping has improved and physical signs of anxiety are reduced.
    3. The patient is able to work around machinery.
    4. Physical signs of anxiety such as pacing have increased.

16. Why are patients who experience anxiety with other conditions treated with benzodiazepine therapy? **(227)**

1. Because generally the patient will not tolerate fluoxetine or any other SSRI.
2. Because the patient will respond most readily with a reduction in anxiety.
3. Because response to behavior therapy works better than drugs.
4. Because the patient will not have any recurrence of symptoms after treatment.

17. Nurses need to teach patients taking hydroxyzine therapy for anxiety to report which symptoms that should be monitored? **(230)**
    1. Dry mouth
    2. Morning hangover
    3. Reduction in anxiety
    4. Slurred speech and dizziness

18. What information does the nurse include during patient teaching for antianxiety therapy? **(225)**
    1. "You may take this medication while operating machinery."
    2. "Therapeutic effects of the drug take 4-6 weeks to occur."
    3. "When discontinuing the medication, there is no need to reduce the dose gradually."
    4. "Notify your healthcare provider if hangover symptoms persist, because the dose may need to be reduced or the medication changed."

19. Which drugs may increase the toxic effects of benzodiazepines? *(Select all that apply.)* **(228)**
    1. Antihistamines
    2. Alcohol
    3. Analgesics
    4. Beta blockers
    5. SSRIs

Discuss psychological and physiologic drug dependence.

20. When a patient is experiencing withdrawal symptoms from long-term use of benzodiazepines, the nurse assesses for which effect ? *(Select all that apply.)* **(227)**
    1. Tremors
    2. Restlessness
    3. Worsening of anxiety
    4. Decreased heart rate
    5. Auditory hypersensitivity

21. The nurse is assessing a patient before administering buspirone (BuSpar). Which finding would the nurse call the prescriber about to determine the appropriateness of the drug? **(228)**
    1. Slurred speech
    2. Insomnia
    3. Nervousness
    4. Dizziness

22. Psychological and physiologic dependence may occur in patients taking which drug? **(227)**
    1. buspirone
    2. hydroxyzine
    3. fluvoxamine
    4. diazepam

Drugs Used for Depressive and Bipolar Disorders

chapter

16

Answer Key: Textbook page references are provided as a guide for answering these questions. A complete answer key is provided to your instructor.

MATCHING

Match the definition on the right with the term on the left.

Term

1. _____ depression
2. _____ mania
3. _____ cyclothymia
4. _____ euphoria
5. _____ grandiose delusions
6. _____ dysthymia
7. _____ labile mood
8. _____ suicidal ideation

Definition

a. the delusion that one has great talents or special powers
b. a milder form of bipolar illness characterized by episodes of depression and hypomania
c. a rapid shift in mood toward anger and irritability
d. a persistent, reduced ability to experience pleasure in life's usual activities
e. a heightened mood
f. thoughts about killing oneself
g. a mood disturbance characterized by elation and euphoria
h. a chronic form of depression with ongoing symptoms lasting for at least 2 years

REVIEW QUESTIONS

Scenario: A 78-year-old patient came into the clinic complaining of insomnia and lack of motivation to do daily activities, which has been increasing in occurrence for the last several months.

Describe the essential components of the baseline assessment of a patient with depression or bipolar disorder.

9. What are characteristic symptoms found in a person experiencing depression? *(Select all that apply.)* **(233)**
   1. Sadness
   2. Slowed thinking
   3. Extreme changes in mood
   4. Inability to concentrate
   5. Increase in appetite
10. The patient in the scenario is likely suffering from which disorder? **(233)**
    1. Mania
    2. Depression
    3. Bipolar disorder
    4. Labile mood

11. The nurse is assessing a patient who is being started on imipramine (Tofranil) and is reviewing the basic components of the assessment for mood disorders, which include asking the patient about: *(Select all that apply.)* **(236-237)**
    1. hygiene habits.
    2. thoughts of death.
    3. job expectations.
    4. interpersonal relationships.
    5. history of mood disorders.
12. Bipolar disorder is characterized by what symptoms? **(233)**
    1. Pacing, hand-wringing, and outbursts of shouting
    2. Alternating episodes of mania and depression
    3. Slowed thinking, confusion, and poor memory
    4. Episodes of mania and depression separated by intervals without mood disturbances
13. What are symptoms of acute mania occurring during the manic phase of bipolar disorder? *(Select all that apply.)* **(234)**
    1. Paranoia
    2. Heightened mood
    3. Increased energy
    4. Increased need for sleep
    5. Abrupt onset of symptoms that escalate over several days

14. What do patients experiencing the manic phase of bipolar disorder generally do? *(234)*
    1. Develop a stable mood during this phase.
    2. Will not develop psychotic symptoms.
    3. Recognize the symptoms of illness in themselves.
    4. Will not recognize the symptoms of illness in themselves.

Identify the premedication assessments that are necessary before the administration of MAOIs, SNRIs, TCAs, and antimanic agents.

15. When patients experience the physiologic manifestations of depression such as sleep disturbance, change in appetite, loss of energy, fatigue, or palpitations, they can expect to have some relief from these symptoms after starting on antidepressants within what timeframe? *(239, 242, 245)*
    1. Within the first three doses of starting therapy
    2. After the second day of starting therapy
    3. After the second week of starting therapy
    4. After the sixth week of starting therapy

16. What are important nursing interventions to implement when caring for patients with mood disorders? *(Select all that apply.)* *(237)*
    1. Provide an environment of acceptance.
    2. Remain calm, direct, and firm when providing care.
    3. Expect the patient to be unable to make decisions.
    4. Patients in the manic phase need to be with people.
    5. Provide an opportunity for the patient to express feelings.

17. The treatment of mood disorders requires nonpharmacologic and pharmacologic therapy, and may include what other therapies? *(Select all that apply.)* *(237)*
    1. Interpersonal therapy
    2. Electroconvulsive therapy
    3. Psychodynamic therapy
    4. Cognitive-behavioral therapy
    5. Electrolysis therapy

18. The premedication assessment that nurses perform for TCAs includes which nursing implication? *(Select all that apply.)* *(245)*
    1. Checking for a history of seizures
    2. Obtaining the patient's height and weight
    3. Determining if there is any history of dysrhythmias
    4. Taking the patient's blood pressure and reporting hypotension
    5. Noting constituency of the patient's stools to watch for constipation

19. The medication assessment that nurses perform for antimanic agents includes which nursing intervention? *(Select all that apply.)* *(251-252)*
    1. Weighing the patient weekly
    2. Obtaining baseline blood pressures supine, sitting, and standing
    3. Administering the antimanic agent on an empty stomach
    4. Obtaining laboratory tests such as electrolytes, blood glucose, and blood urea nitrogen (BUN)
    5. Monitoring lithium levels once or twice weekly during the start of therapy

Compare the mechanism of action of selective serotonin reuptake inhibitors (SSRIs) with that of other antidepressant agents.

20. SSRIs act by which mechanism of action? *(242)*
    1. By an unknown exact mechanism of action
    2. By blocking the destruction of serotonin
    3. By inhibiting the reuptake of serotonin
    4. By inhibiting the degradation of serotonin

21. SSRIs are the most widely used class of antidepressants because they have been shown to be effective and also are considered to: *(242)*
    1. be safe for children.
    2. be less costly.
    3. have no anticholinergic adverse effects.
    4. be more effective than other antidepressants.

22. SSRIs are being studied to identify if these agents can successfully be used to treat which other disorders? *(Select all that apply.)* *(242)*
    1. Autism
    2. Anorexia nervosa
    3. Panic disorders
    4. Diabetic retinopathy
    5. Menopausal symptoms

23. Which SSRI is approved for treatment of depression in children and adolescents? *(242)*
    1. sertraline (Zoloft)
    2. fluoxetine (Prozac)
    3. paroxetine (Paxil)
    4. fluvoxamine (Luvox)

24. SSRIs have an advantage over tricyclic antidepressants because they do not have which effect? *(242)*
    1. They do not cause insomnia or restlessness.
    2. They do not require suicidal precautions to be in place.
    3. They do not take 2-4 weeks of therapy to obtain the therapeutic effect.
    4. They do not cause anticholinergic and cardiovascular adverse effects compared to tricyclic antidepressants.

Cite the common adverse effects that may develop for patients who are taking monoamine oxidase inhibitors (MAOIs).

25. When patients are taking MAOIs, the nurse needs to include which instructions for patients? *(Select all that apply.)* *(242)*
    1. How to limit tyramine-containing foods in their diet
    2. The importance of not discontinuing the drug abruptly
    3. To avoid taking the divided dose later than 8 PM
    4. Dividing the dose to prevent drug-induced insomnia
    5. Avoiding the drugs known to cause drug interactions

26. When patients are taking the MAOI selegiline (Emsam), the nurse needs to assess for which adverse effect? *(239)*
    1. Vomiting and diarrhea
    2. Dizziness and weakness
    3. Therapeutic serum levels
    4. Decreased sedation

27. The nurse was instructing a diabetic patient who was starting on the MAOI isocarboxazid (Marplan) regarding precautions to use, and realized further education was needed after the patient made which statement? *(242)*
    1. "Since I have to take insulin, I will need to adjust my doses while I take this drug."
    2. "As I understand it, I can stop taking my insulin since this drug will cause hypoglycemia."
    3. "I get it; I need to carefully monitor my blood sugar while I am on this drug."
    4. "I will need to carefully determine what foods I can eat while on this drug."

Cite the common adverse effects that may develop for patients who are taking serotonin-norepinephrine reuptake inhibitors (SNRIs).

28. What are nursing implications for patients on SNRI therapy? *(Select all that apply.)* *(244)*
    1. Recognizing improvement may take up 2-4 weeks
    2. Understanding that depression will be alleviated entirely with therapy
    3. Knowing that suicide precautions should be maintained during first several weeks of therapy
    4. Educating the patients regarding common adverse effects such as constipation
    5. Tapering venlafaxine over 2 weeks if taken for longer than 6 weeks when discontinuing the drug

29. What do nurses need to assess for in patients prior to starting therapy with the SNRI duloxetine (Cymbalta)? *(Select all that apply.)* *(244)*
    1. GI symptoms
    2. Glaucoma
    3. Insomnia
    4. Hypertension
    5. Thyroid disorders

30. Nurses need to explain to patients that they cannot work with machinery or operate a motor vehicle if they develop which adverse effect from SNRIs? *(244)*
    1. Insomnia
    2. Nausea or anorexia
    3. Dizziness or drowsiness
    4. Restlessness, anxiety, or agitation

Cite the common adverse effects that may develop for patients who are taking tricyclic antidepressants (TCAs).

31. When patients are taking TCAs for depression, what is the most important baseline parameter the nurse needs to assess? *(245)*
    1. Pulse
    2. Weight
    3. Temperature
    4. Blood pressure in supine and sitting positions

32. Primary outcomes expected from TCAs include elevated mood and reduction of symptoms of depression, and TCAs can also be used for the treatment of which conditions? *(Select all that apply.)* *(245)*
    1. Anxiety
    2. Glaucoma
    3. Hypertension
    4. Enuresis in children
    5. Obsessive-compulsive disorders

33. Selected TCAs are also used to treat which other disorders? *(Select all that apply.)* *(245)*
    1. Cancer pain
    2. Arthritic pain
    3. Phantom limb pain
    4. Premenstrual symptoms
    5. Menopause symptoms

Cite the common adverse effects that may develop for patients who are taking lithium.

34. What drug is most commonly used to treat the manic phase of bipolar disorder? *(251)*
    1. citalopram
    2. lithium carbonate
    3. duloxetine
    4. venlafaxine

35. When the antimanic agent lithium is used for patients with bipolar disorder, the nurse educates the patient and family on which ways to prevent toxicity? *(Select all that apply.)* **(252)**
    1. "Lithium needs to be taken with food or milk."
    2. "The full therapeutic effect of this drug often requires 21-30 days."
    3. "You will need to maintain a normal dietary intake of sodium with adequate water."
    4. "You will need to monitor your lithium levels once or twice weekly during the start of this therapy."
    5. "You need to report immediately any persistent vomiting and diarrhea, as these are signs of toxicity."

36. The nurse needs to assess for early signs of lithium toxicity, which include: *(Select all that apply.)* **(252)**
    1. lethargy.
    2. increased appetite.
    3. nausea and vomiting.
    4. speech difficulties.
    5. muscle twitching and tremors.

Drugs Used for Psychoses

Answer Key: Textbook page references are provided as a guide for answering these questions. A complete answer key is provided to your instructor.

MATCHING

Match the term on the right with the definition on the left.

Definition

1. _____ spasmodic movements of muscle groups

2. _____ a syndrome of persistent and involuntary hyperkinetic abnormal movements

3. _____ tremors, muscle rigidity, mask-like expressions, shuffling gait, and loss or weakness of motor function

4. _____ a syndrome of anxiety and restlessness, and associated pacing, rocking, and an inability to sit or stand in one place for extended periods

5. _____ term that applies to someone who is out of touch with reality

6. _____ adverse effects of antipsychotic medications associated with nonadherence to therapy

7. _____ false sensory perceptions, experienced as real to the patient

Term

a. pseudoparkinsonian symptoms
b. hallucinations
c. tardive dyskinesia
d. akathisia
e. extrapyramidal symptoms
f. dystonias
g. psychosis

REVIEW QUESTIONS

Scenario: A 45-year-old male patient was admitted to the inpatient psychiatric unit for further evaluation and treatment after he was found by his family to be babbling incoherently and rapidly pacing in his apartment. He has a history of schizoid affective disorder and had not taken his medications lately.

Identify the signs and symptoms of psychotic behavior.

8. The patient is said to be suffering from psychosis when which of these symptoms are present? *(Select all that apply.)* **(255)**
   1. Insomnia
   2. Delusions
   3. Hallucinations
   4. Orthostatic hypotension
   5. Disorganized thinking

9. A patient in the emergency department tells the nurse that he is the creator of the universe. What does the nurse suspect that this patient is experiencing? **(255)**
   1. Delusions
   2. Hallucinations
   3. Change of affect
   4. Disorganized thinking

10. Target symptoms are critical monitoring parameters used to assess changes in the patient's status and his or her response to medications. Which are examples of target symptoms? *(Select all that apply.)* **(256)**
    1. Weight gain
    2. Loose associations
    3. Substance abuse
    4. Frequency and type of agitation
    5. Degree of suspiciousness

Describe the major indications for the use of antipsychotic agents.

11. Underlying disorders which may cause psychosis may not necessitate the use of antipsychotic agents, but rather treatment of which disorder? *(Select all that apply.)* **(255)**
    1. Infections
    2. Endocrine disorders
    3. Schizophrenia
    4. Bipolar disorders
    5. Metabolic disturbances

12. Psychotic symptoms common with which mood disorders necessitate the patient being started on an antipsychotic agent? *(Select all that apply.)* **(255)**
    1. Anorexia
    2. Schizophrenia
    3. Bipolar disorder
    4. Major depression
    5. Obsessive-compulsive disorder

13. In the teaching for the patient in the scenario, the nurse should include that taking antipsychotic agents may cause dystonic reactions that: **(261)**
    1. usually last for 1 week.
    2. may not be responsive to treatment.
    3. occur most often in females.
    4. occur most often in the first 72 hours of therapy.

Discuss the antipsychotic medications that are used for the treatment of psychoses.

14. First-generation antipsychotic agents such as the phenothiazines are thought to have which mechanism of action? **(257)**
    1. Block serotonin reuptake inhibitors
    2. Block the serotonin receptors
    3. Block dopamine in the brain
    4. Release serotonin at the receptor sites

15. The second-generation or atypical antipsychotic agents are thought to have which mechanism of action? **(257)**
    1. Block serotonin reuptake inhibitors
    2. Block the dopamine and serotonin receptors
    3. Block dopamine in the brain
    4. Release serotonin at the receptor sites

16. Atypical antipsychotic agents are most commonly used because they tend to be more effective in relieving negative symptoms. These agents include which medications? *(Select all that apply.)* **(259)**
    1. haloperidol (Haldol)
    2. risperidone (Risperdal)
    3. quetiapine (Seroquel)
    4. aripiprazole (Abilify)
    5. ziprasidone (Geodon)

Identify the common adverse effects that are observed with the use of antipsychotic medications.

17. The nurse will discuss with the patient in the scenario who is taking an antipsychotic drug that he may experience which adverse effects? *(Select all that apply.)* **(266)**
    1. Seizures
    2. Hypoglycemia
    3. Weight loss
    4. Tardive dyskinesia
    5. Orthostatic hypotension

18. Patients taking antipsychotic medications may experience which common adverse effects? *(Select all that apply.)* **(266)**
    1. Diarrhea
    2. Chronic fatigue
    3. Dry mouth
    4. Blurred vision
    5. Urinary retention

19. A patient has been started on the atypical antipsychotic clozapine (Clozaril) for bipolar disorder. For the first 6 months of therapy, which lab result is most important for the nurse to monitor? **(266)**
    1. Red blood cell counts
    2. White blood cell counts
    3. Blood glucose
    4. Thyroid-stimulating hormone

Drugs Used for Seizure Disorders

Answer Key: Textbook page references are provided as a guide for answering these questions. A complete answer key is provided to your instructor.

MATCHING

Match the term on the right with the definition on the left.

Definition

1. _____ a rapidly recurring generalized seizure that does not allow the patient to regain normal function between seizures

2. _____ seizures that begin in a localized area in one hemisphere of the brain

3. _____ recovery phase of flaccid paralysis and sleep

4. _____ bilaterally symmetric jerks alternating with the relaxation of the extremities

5. _____ a sudden loss of muscle tone, or drop attack

6. _____ a diagnosis applied to patients with chronic and recurrent seizures

7. _____ lightning-like repetitive contractions of the voluntary muscles of the face, trunk, and extremities

8. _____ a back-and-forth movement of the eyeballs on a horizontal plane

9. _____ intense muscular contractions; patients may fall, lose consciousness, and lie rigid

Term

a. epilepsy
b. nystagmus
c. postictal state
d. tonic phase
e. clonic phase
f. status epilepticus
g. atonic seizure
h. myoclonic seizure
i. focal seizures

REVIEW QUESTIONS

Scenario: A 32-year-old female patient was admitted to the hospital following an episode of a generalized seizure witnessed by her husband.

Identify the different types of seizure disorders.

10. During which types of seizures is it not uncommon for patients to lose their balance and fall with no loss of consciousness? *(270)*
    1. Tonic-clonic and myoclonic
    2. Myoclonic and atonic
    3. Atonic and tonic-clonic
    4. Absence and myoclonic

11. When monitoring a patient during a seizure, the nurse knows that atonic seizures manifest as what? *(270)*
    1. Intense muscular contractions
    2. Bilateral jerks alternating with relaxation of the extremities
    3. A sudden loss of muscle tone, occurring in short attacks
    4. Lightning-like repetitive contractions of the muscles of the face

12. Which type of seizure is considered a medical emergency and prompt treatment is necessary to prevent nerve damage and death? *(270)*
    1. Myoclonic seizures
    2. Tonic-clonic seizures
    3. Absence seizures
    4. Status epilepticus

13. Seizures are divided into which classifications? *(269)*
    1. Full seizures and partial seizures
    2. Generalized seizures and partial seizures
    3. Grand mal seizures and petit mal seizures
    4. Generalized convulsive seizures and generalized nonconvulsive seizures

Identify nursing interventions during the management of seizure activity.

14. The nurse needs to educate the patient in the scenario on what to expect from the seizure medications, as well as which common adverse effects that may occur? *(Select all that apply.)* *(276, 278, 287)*
    1. Drowsiness
    2. Dizziness
    3. Orthostatic hypotension
    4. Blood dyscrasias
    5. Nausea and vomiting

15. Which action does the nurse take when working with a patient experiencing a seizure? *(272)*
    1. Restrains the patient and places a tongue blade in the patient's mouth
    2. Medicates the patient immediately and observes for signs of recovery
    3. Asks the family to leave the room if present, and calmly waits outside the room for the seizure to stop
    4. Once the patient enters into the recovery phase, turns him or her slightly onto the side to allow secretions to drain from the mouth

16. The nurse is discussing the diagnosis of epilepsy to parents of a 5-year-old child who had been recently diagnosed with tonic-clonic seizures. Which statement by the parents indicates that the nurse needs to educate further? *(270)*
    1. "These seizures will be outgrown later in life."
    2. "Seizures are grouped into two types, generalized and partial."
    3. "*Epilepsy* is the general term meaning that the seizures are chronic."
    4. "The tonic-clonic seizures that were diagnosed have a recovery stage."

17. Nurses need to document what is happening to a patient during a seizure and include which information regarding the seizure? *(Select all that apply.)* *(272)*
    1. Duration of the seizure
    2. Progression of symptoms
    3. Onset or possible causal factor
    4. State of consciousness
    5. Which hemisphere of the brain is being affected

18. The nurse is teaching the patient in the scenario about the use of phenytoin (Dilantin) for seizure control. What does the nurse tell the patient about taking oral contraceptives with this medication? *(277)*
    1. "You will not be able to become pregnant because of the phenytoin therapy."
    2. "There are no contraindications for using these two drugs together."
    3. "Dilantin therapy should be stopped if you experience spotting or bleeding."
    4. "An alternative form of birth control should be used when taking phenytoin with oral contraceptives."

Cite the desired therapeutic outcomes from antiepileptic agents used for seizure disorders.

19. When administering antiepileptic agents to patients, the nurse knows that the therapeutic outcomes include what? *(Select all that apply.)* *(270)*
    1. A reduced frequency of seizures
    2. A reduction in any injury from seizure activity
    3. Minimal adverse effects from therapy
    4. A reduction in tension and stress
    5. An alleviation of any seizure activity

20. Which drugs are often used for the initial treatment of a newly diagnosed seizure disorder such as the patient in the scenario? *(Select all that apply.)* *(271)*
    1. lorazepam (Ativan)
    2. gabapentin (Neurontin)
    3. lamotrigine (Lamictal)
    4. topiramate (Topamax)
    5. levetiracetam (Keppra)

21. When the patient is started on an antiepileptic drug, the nurse needs to closely monitor for which adverse effect that may occur as early as 1 week or as late as several months? *(271)*
    1. Suicidal ideation
    2. Refractory seizures
    3. Increased use of caffeine-containing products
    4. Halitosis, requiring increase frequency of oral hygiene

Identify the drug classes used to treat seizure disorders.

22. Benzodiazepines are used for the treatment of seizures because they are thought to have what effect? *(273)*
    1. Prevent reuptake of GABA
    2. Cause the destruction of GABA
    3. Prevent the breakdown of dopamine
    4. Enhance the effects of gamma-aminobutyric acid (GABA)

23. Succinimides are drugs that are used to decrease the frequency of seizures by which mechanism of action? *(277)*
    1. Enhancing the effects of GABA
    2. Blocking the reuptake of norepinephrine
    3. Preventing the breakdown of dopamine
    4. Reducing the current in the T-type calcium channels
24. The miscellaneous antiepileptic agent carbamazepine (Tegretol) works by which mechanism of action? *(278)*
    1. By decreasing the effectiveness of GABA
    2. By blocking the reuptake of norepinephrine
    3. By increasing the effectiveness of GABA
    4. By increasing the rate of dopamine being released
25. The anticonvulsant lamotrigine, unrelated to other antiepileptic medications, is thought to act by blocking voltage-sensitive sodium and calcium channels, and is part of which class of drugs? *(280)*
    1. Sulfonamides
    2. Phenyltriazine
    3. Succinimides
    4. Pyrrolidines

Describe the neurologic assessment performed on patients taking antiepileptic agents to monitor for common and serious adverse effects.

26. Patients who are diabetic and taking hydantoins need to be educated on the risk of which complication? *(276)*
    1. Developing oral thrush
    2. Decreased effectiveness of hydantoin
    3. Hyperglycemia with hydantoin therapy
    4. Increased frequency of hypoglycemia
27. When patients are on antacids and hydantoins, they should be told that the antacid will have what effect? *(277)*
    1. Decrease the therapeutic effect of phenytoin
    2. Increase the therapeutic effect of phenytoin
    3. Increase the level of hydantoin in the blood, causing toxicity
    4. Decrease the therapeutic effects of the antacid
28. The nurse assessing the patient in the scenario who is starting on topiramate (Topamax) knows to monitor for which common adverse effects? *(Select all that apply.) (287)*
    1. Sedation
    2. Dizziness
    3. Drowsiness
    4. Constipation
    5. Increased sweating

Drugs Used for Pain Management

Answer Key: Textbook page references are provided as a guide for answering these questions. A complete answer key is provided to your instructor.

MATCHING

Match the definition on the right with the term on the left.

Term

1. _____ pain experience
2. _____ pain perception
3. _____ pain threshold
4. _____ pain tolerance

Definition

a. the point at which an individual first acknowledges or interprets a sensation of pain
b. an individual's awareness of the feeling or sensation of pain
c. the individual's ability to endure pain
d. an unpleasant sensation that is highly subjective and influenced by sensory, emotional, and cultural factors

REVIEW QUESTIONS

Scenario: A patient recovering from a recent fall that resulted in broken vertebrae and the need for a 'turtle shell' for back support was talking with a nurse about pain control.

Describe the pain assessment used for patients receiving opiate agonists.

5. The nurse in the scenario is discussing various pain management options with the patient and realizes more education is needed when the patient makes which statement? *(295)*
   1. "I will need to limit the amount of exercise I get while taking codeine."
   2. "One of the goals I have for pain relief is to be able to sleep at least 6 hours without waking up."
   3. "I know I need to eat a well-balanced diet and drink plenty of water while taking codeine."
   4. "I understand I can use other measures to relieve pain in addition to taking this codeine, like a heating pad."

6. For patients taking opiate agonists, the nurse needs to monitor the patient for signs of which adverse effects? *(Select all that apply.) (306)*
   1. Diarrhea
   2. Hyperglycemia
   3. Urinary retention
   4. Respiratory depression
   5. Confusion or disorientation

7. When determining if the patient has pain, the nurse needs to assess which components of the pain assessment? *(Select all that apply.) (299)*
   1. The location of pain
   2. The rating on a pain scale
   3. The duration of pain
   4. The quality of pain
   5. The last time no pain was felt

Differentiate among the properties of opiate agonists, opiate partial agonists, and opiate antagonists.

8. The nurse understands that opiate agonists interact with receptors to stimulate a response of pain relief, whereas partial agonists may do what? *(307)*
   1. Block any response
   2. Induce a stupor or sleep
   3. Stimulate a response, but may inhibit other responses
   4. Induce withdrawal symptoms if any opiate agonist has been given

9. What is the mechanism of action for opiate antagonists? *(309)*
   1. To block the effects of any euphoric high
   2. To stimulate a response of pain relief
   3. To reverse the depressant effects of any opiate agonist
   4. To stimulate a response, but may inhibit other responses

10. The nurse knows which is true about the use of the transdermal opioid analgesic fentanyl (Duragesic)? *(305)*
    1. Fentanyl is only used for acute pain.
    2. Fentanyl patches provide relief for up to 72 hours.
    3. No other analgesics may be used concurrently with fentanyl.
    4. Approximately 2 hours are required for the initial patch of medication to reach a steady blood level.

Cite the common adverse effects of opiate agonists.

11. The patient in the scenario is receiving opiate agonists for pain control. Which adverse effect does the nurse report to the healthcare provider? *(Select all that apply.) (306-307)*
    1. Dry mouth
    2. Lightheadedness
    3. Respiratory rate of 7
    4. Urinary retention
    5. Daily bowel movements

12. Which common adverse effect can usually be treated by diet and stool softeners? *(306)*
    1. Constipation
    2. Urinary retention
    3. Respiratory depression
    4. Orthostatic hypotension

13. What should the nurse instruct patients who report lightheadedness and dizziness after the first dose of hydromorphone (Dilaudid) to do? *(306)*
    1. Remain lying down.
    2. Increase the amount of whole-grain products in their diet.
    3. Report this effect to the healthcare provider for further evaluation.
    4. Sit up quickly and stand after 30 seconds of sitting to relieve symptoms.

14. If an opiate partial agonist (nalbuphine) is administered to a patient who is addicted to the opiate agonist (oxycodone), what must the nurse assess for? *(308)*
    1. Constipation
    2. Hypotension
    3. Elevated WBCs
    4. Withdrawal symptoms

15. What drugs are antidotes for opiate agonists and opiate partial agonists? *(308)*
    1. Naloxone (Evzio) and pentazocine (Talwin)
    2. Naltrexone (ReVia) and nalbuphine (Nubain)
    3. Naloxone (Evzio) and naltrexone (ReVia)
    4. Naltrexone (ReVia) and butorphanol (Stadol)

16. When are opiate partial agonists effective in relieving pain? *(307)*
    1. For people who have recently taken opiate agonists
    2. After opiate agonists are no longer effective
    3. For patients after surgery in conjunction with opiate agonists
    4. In cases without prior administration of opiate agonists

Describe the three pharmacologic effects of salicylates.

17. Salicylates are known to have which pharmacologic properties? *(313)*
    1. Antiepileptic, antiplatelet, and antiinflammatory
    2. Analgesic, antiplatelet, and antacid
    3. Analgesic, antipyretic, and antiinflammatory
    4. Antiinflammatory, antipyretic, and antacid

18. Salicylates are used for which conditions? *(Select all that apply.) (313)*
    1. Reduce fever from infections
    2. Relief of inflammation from rheumatoid arthritis
    3. Prevent the symptoms of withdrawal from opiates
    4. Reduce the risk of recurrent TIA or stroke
    5. Reduce the risk of myocardial infarction

19. Salicylates work by inhibiting prostaglandins, which when activated cause what effect? *(Select all that apply.) (313)*
    1. The platelets to aggregate
    2. Sensitization of the pain receptors that cause pain
    3. Elevation of body temperature
    4. Mental sluggishness and sedation
    5. Signs and symptoms of inflammation

List the common and serious adverse effects and drug interactions associated with salicylates.

20. A patient has been taking an oral hypoglycemic agent and is being started on salicylate therapy for pain management. What does the nurse anticipate will happen when these two types of drugs are taken together? *(317)*
    1. The patient will need to switch to subcutaneous insulin therapy for the duration of the salicylate therapy.
    2. The oral hypoglycemic agent will potentiate the effect of the salicylate and increase the chance of salicylate toxicity.
    3. The dose of the oral hypoglycemic agent will be doubled while the patient is on salicylate therapy.
    4. Salicylates may enhance the hypoglycemic effects of oral hypoglycemic agents; therefore, the dose may need to be reduced.

21. Salicylates should not be used in children because of which associated risk? *(313)*
    1. Overdose
    2. Reye's syndrome
    3. Toxic response
    4. Respiratory depression
22. Salicylates should not be given when patients have which conditions? *(Select all that apply.) (313)*
    1. Peptic ulcers
    2. Glaucoma
    3. Liver disease
    4. Coagulation disorders
    5. Previous myocardial infarctions
23. When comparing the therapeutic effects of NSAIDs to acetaminophen (Tylenol), the nurse knows that both are very good antipyretic and analgesic agents; however what is the difference? *(312)*
    1. Acetaminophen has antiplatelet effects.
    2. NSAIDs have antiplatelet effects.
    3. Acetaminophen has no antiinflammatory effect.
    4. NSAIDs have no effect on prostaglandins.
24. What are the primary therapeutic outcomes expected from acetaminophen (Tylenol)? *(312)*
    1. To reduce inflammation and pain
    2. To reduce pain and fever
    3. To relieve pain and heartburn
    4. To improve circulation and nasal congestion
25. What are the three NSAIDs available over the counter? *(317)*
    1. Meloxicam (Mobic), indomethacin (Indocin), ketorolac (Apo-Ketorolac)
    2. Ibuprofen (Advil), naproxen (Aleve), ketaprofen (Apo-Keto)
    3. Diclofenac (Cataflam), oxaprozin (Daypro), celecoxib (Celebrex)
    4. Sulindac (Apo-Sulin), diclofenac (Cataflam), indomethacin (Indocin)
26. The nurse is explaining to the patient in the scenario that the active ingredients in Anacin include what drugs? *(316)*
    1. Aspirin and caffeine
    2. Aspirin and hydrocodone
    3. Acetaminophen and aspirin
    4. Acetaminophen and caffeine
27. The nurse is instructing a patient who is allergic to acetaminophen (Tylenol) on the use of which combination product that would be safe to take? *(316)*
    1. Fioricet
    2. Percocet 7.5
    3. Percodan
    4. Excedrin Extra Strength
28. A nurse was explaining to the patient in the scenario the difference between Norco and Vicodin, and makes which correct statement? *(316)*
    1. "Norco has aspirin and Vicodin has Tylenol."
    2. "Norco has more hydromorphone in it than Vicodin."
    3. "Norco has more hydrocodone in it than Vicodin."
    4. "There is no difference; they are just made by different drug companies."

Identify opiate antagonists and expected therapeutic outcomes to monitor.

29. Emergency service personnel across the nation now carry the opiate antagonist naloxone (Evzio) for cases of what? *(319)*
    1. Acute hemorrhage
    2. Food poisoning
    3. Acute anaphylaxis by bee stings
    4. Potential overdoses of opiates
30. What effect does the opiate antagonist naloxone (Evzio) have? *(Select all that apply.) (309)*
    1. Increase GI motility
    2. Reverse respiratory depression
    3. Decrease the incidence of allergic reactions
    4. Activate the clotting cascade in cases of acute hemorrhage
    5. Reverse CNS depression caused by excessive doses of opiate agonists
31. Which opiate antagonist can be given orally? *(311)*
    1. Naloxone
    2. Naltrexone
    3. Naproxen
    4. Nabumetone

Introduction to Cardiovascular Disease and Metabolic Syndrome

chapter
20

Answer Key: Textbook page references are provided as a guide for answering these questions. A complete answer key is provided to your instructor.

MATCHING
Match the term on the right with the definition on the left.

Definitions

1. _____ abnormalities in the electrical conduction pathways of the heart

2. _____ a narrowing or obstruction of the arteries of the heart

3. _____ an obstruction or rupture of blood vessels in the brain

4. _____ involves disorders of the blood vessels of the arms and legs

5. _____ an increase in the pressure with which blood circulates through the arteries

Terms

a. hypertension
b. dysrhythmias
c. coronary artery disease
d. peripheral vascular disease
e. stroke

REVIEW QUESTIONS

Scenario: A 42-year-old male patient discussed with the nurse the need for exercising, as he had previously indicated that he rarely exercises. The nurse was asking questions designed to get him to think about why he does not exercise and what some of his beliefs are about this, as he was obese and just diagnosed with hypertension.

Identify the major risk factors for the development of metabolic syndrome.

6. The nurse will explain to the patient in the scenario the risk factors that he needs to consider that may lead to the development of metabolic syndrome, which include what factors? *(Select all that apply.)* *(322)*
   1. Obesity
   2. Diabetes
   3. Hypertension
   4. Active lifestyle
   5. Stressful occupation

7. The risk factor of lower levels of HDL cholesterol is important to consider for developing metabolic syndrome because it can lead to: *(322)*
   1. diabetes.
   2. hypertension.
   3. heart attack or stroke.
   4. insulin resistance syndrome.

8. Examples of cardiovascular disorders that are attributed to the narrowing or obstruction of the arteries of the heart include which? *(Select all that apply.)* *(322)*
   1. Stroke
   2. Hypertension
   3. Angina pectoris
   4. Myocardial infarction
   5. Peripheral vascular disease

9. In addition to type 2 diabetes and heart disease, which other consequences are associated with metabolic syndrome? *(Select all that apply.)* *(322)*
   1. Renal disease
   2. Liver disease
   3. Obstructive sleep apnea
   4. Cognitive decline in older adults
   5. Polycystic ovary syndrome

10. Which are examples of peripheral vascular disease involving disorders of the blood vessels of the arms and legs? *(Select all that apply.)* *(321)*
    1. Stroke
    2. Diabetes
    3. Myocardial infarction
    4. Obstructive arterial disease
    5. Deep vein thrombosis

Discuss the importance of lifestyle modification in the management of metabolic syndrome.

11. Which modification should the nurse encourage when teaching health promotion to the patient in the scenario with metabolic syndrome? (*Select all that apply.*) (323)
    1. Smoking cessation
    2. Weight reduction
    3. Vigorous exercise
    4. Stress reduction
    5. Dietary modification

12. When teaching the patient in the scenario about metabolic syndrome, the nurse discusses ways to promote weight loss and increased physical activity by which methods? (*Select all that apply.*) (323)
    1. Adopting the DASH diet
    2. Reducing the number of calories eaten
    3. Exercising at the same time of day consistently
    4. Getting 60 minutes of moderate-intensity physical activity twice a week
    5. Dietary fat should be unsaturated, and simple sugars should be reduced

13. What are some of the characteristics of a sedentary lifestyle that contribute to obesity and the development of metabolic syndrome? (*Select all that apply.*) (323)
    1. Work-related stress
    2. Labor-saving devices
    3. Remote control devices
    4. Genetic predisposition
    5. Entertainment through television and computers

Explain the treatment goals for type 2 diabetes management, lipid management, and hypertension management.

14. Which drug classes are used to treat type 2 diabetes mellitus associated with metabolic syndrome because they will stimulate the beta cells of the pancreas to release more insulin? (326)
    1. Sulfonylureas and meglitinides
    2. Meglitinides and thiazolidinediones
    3. Thiazolidinediones and alpha-glucosidase inhibitors
    4. Sulfonylureas and thiazolidinediones

15. Treatment of dyslipidemia is generally to lower the triglycerides and LDL cholesterol and raise the HDL cholesterol and includes which drug class? (*Select all that apply.*) (326)
    1. Statins
    2. Thiazide diuretics
    3. Calcium channel blockers
    4. Fibric acid derivatives
    5. Alpha-glucosidase inhibitors

16. When teaching the patient in the scenario with metabolic syndrome about the importance of weight loss and a healthy diet, the nurse includes which statement? (325)
    1. "Olive oil is an example of the type of 'good' fat you may eat."
    2. "Most of the dietary fat you consume should be saturated."
    3. "You must limit the amount of protein you eat to 2 ounces once a day."
    4. "Restrict the total amount of fat you consume each day to approximately 45% of your total calories."

17. The treatment for hypertension when changes in diet and exercise do not produce acceptable reduction in blood pressure include which drug class? (*Select all that apply.*) (325-326)
    1. Analgesics
    2. Thiazide diuretics
    3. Calcium channel blockers
    4. Alpha-glucosidase inhibitors
    5. Angiotensin-converting enzyme inhibitors

Discuss the drug management of the underlying diseases used by patients with metabolic syndrome.

18. The overall treatment goals for metabolic syndrome include which parameters? (*Select all that apply.*) (325)
    1. LDL of < 100 mg/dL
    2. Hemoglobin A1C levels < 7%
    3. Triglyceride levels of < 150 mg/dL
    4. Fasting blood sugar of < 120 mg/dL
    5. Blood pressure of < 150/90 mm Hg

19. What is recognized as the greatest contributor to a variety of diseases? (321)
    1. Diet
    2. Lifestyle
    3. Medications
    4. Hypertension

20. Which lab values indicate that the general treatment goals for patients with metabolic syndrome are being met? (*Select all that apply.*) (325)
    1. LDL of 140 mg/dL
    2. HDL of 55 mg/dL
    3. Postprandial plasma glucose of 140 mg/dL
    4. Hemoglobin A1C of 5%
    5. Fasting plasma glucose of 118 mg/dL

Drugs Used to Treat Dyslipidemias

Answer Key: Textbook page references are provided as a guide for answering these questions. A complete answer key is provided to your instructor.

MATCHING

Match the term on the right with the definition on the left.

Definition

1. _____ substance essential for synthesizing steroids and bile acids

2. _____ characterized by the accumulation of fatty deposits on the inner walls of blood vessels

3. _____ 90% triglycerides and 5% cholesterol

4. _____ a broad term used to classify patients with high levels of blood fats

5. _____ a precursor to cholesterol

Term

a. hyperlipidemia
b. atherosclerosis
c. triglycerides
d. chylomicrons
e. cholesterol

REVIEW QUESTIONS

Scenario: An obese 58-year-old female patient with hypertension and diabetes was told during a routine checkup that she had elevated levels of cholesterol and needed to be started on antilipid therapy along with diet modification.

Describe atherosclerosis and identify the four major types of lipoproteins.

6. Which condition is characterized by the accumulation of fatty deposits on the inner walls of arteries and arterioles throughout the body that reduce the blood supply to vital organs? *(328)*
   1. Myocardial infarction
   2. Atherosclerosis
   3. Angina pectoris
   4. Cardiac dysrhythmias

7. Which are major treatable causes of coronary artery disease (CAD)? *(Select all that apply.) (328)*
   1. Smoking
   2. Alcoholism
   3. Sedentary lifestyle
   4. Angina pectoris
   5. Type 2 diabetes

8. Which lipoprotein is sometimes referred to as the "good" lipoprotein because high levels indicate that cholesterol is being removed from vascular tissue? *(329)*
   1. IDL
   2. VLDL
   3. LDL
   4. HDL

9. Atherosclerosis impacts the arteries of the heart as well as the arteries and arterioles throughout the body, causing what condition? *(328)*
   1. Urinary retention
   2. Pulmonary hypotension
   3. Peripheral vascular disease
   4. Increased cerebral profusion

10. Lipoproteins are subdivided into five categories based on composition: chylomicrons, very low-density lipoproteins (VLDLs), intermediate-density lipoproteins (IDLs), low-density lipoproteins (LDLs), and high-density lipoproteins (HDLs). The five types differ in relative concentrations of what? *(328)*
    1. Cholesterol, triglycerides, and steroids
    2. Triglycerides, proteins, and amino acids
    3. Cholesterol, protein, and carbohydrates
    4. Triglycerides, cholesterol, and proteins

11. Low levels of HDLs are considered a positive risk factor for the development of what condition? *(329)*
    1. Diabetes
    2. Bleeding disorders
    3. Coronary artery disease
    4. Elevated C-reactive protein levels

Describe the primary approaches to treat lipid disorders.

12. The patient in the scenario came back to the clinic for a checkup after starting atorvastatin (Lipitor) and asked the nurse how the drug works. Which statement by the nurse would be appropriate? *(329)*
    1. "The statins interfere with the absorption of cholesterol from the diet."
    2. "The statins inhibit an enzyme in the pathway to making cholesterol in the liver."
    3. "The statins work best when taken with another antilipid agent to lower your cholesterol level."
    4. "The exact action of statins is unknown, but they are effective agents in reducing cholesterol."

13. In addition to antilipid agents used to treat hyperlipidemias, what other methods are employed for treatment? *(Select all that apply.) (329)*
    1. Diet
    2. Exercise
    3. Weight reduction
    4. Controlling blood pressure
    5. Regular dental checkups

14. Which antilipid agent reduces atherosclerosis by blocking the absorption of cholesterol by the small intestine? *(337)*
    1. simvastatin (Zocor)
    2. omega-3 fatty acids (Lovaza)
    3. ezetimibe (Zetia)
    4. nicotinic acid (Niacin)

15. Which antilipid agent decreases atherosclerosis by combining two omega-3 fatty acids, which act to decrease the synthesis of triglycerides in the liver? *(338)*
    1. ezetimibe (Zetia)
    2. omega-3 fatty acids (Lovaza)
    3. atorvastatin (Lipitor)
    4. gemfibrozil

Determine which antilipid medications are used for cholesterol control and which can be used for triglyceride control.

16. What is now recognized as the greatest contributor to the development of hyperlipidemia? *(329)*
    1. Exercise
    2. Lifestyle
    3. Smoking
    4. Increased vitamin intake

17. The statins are the most potent antilipid agents available with which added benefits that result in decreased heart attacks and stroke? *(Select all that apply.) (334)*
    1. Decreased amounts of HDL
    2. Decreased inflammation
    3. Decreased platelet aggregation
    4. Decreased thrombin formation
    5. Decreased plasma viscosity

18. Which antilipid agents are used to reduce triglyceride levels for patients who have hypertriglyceridemia? *(Select all that apply.) (333, 336)*
    1. Niacin
    2. Statins
    3. Fibric acids
    4. Omega-3 fatty acids
    5. Bile acid–binding resins

Differentiate between how statins work to control lipid levels and how the bile acid resins work to control lipid levels.

19. The nurse instructing the patient in the scenario taking a HMG-CoA reductase inhibitor for the treatment of hyperlipidemia, reminded her to do what? *(336)*
    1. Avoid drinking grapefruit juice.
    2. Have liver function tests monitored every 2 months.
    3. Expect muscle weakness as a common adverse effect.
    4. Take the medication on an empty stomach to increase absorption.

20. When teaching a patient about niacin therapy, the nurse tells the patient to report which adverse effects to the primary healthcare provider? *(Select all that apply.) (334)*
    1. Flushing
    2. Jaundice
    3. Muscle aches
    4. Headaches
    5. Abdominal discomfort

21. A patient taking a bile acid–binding resin for the treatment of dyslipidemia tells the nurse that ever since he began taking the medication, he has experienced bloating and fullness. What does the nurse instruct the patient to do? *(Select all that apply.) (333)*
    1. Limit fluid intake.
    2. Use a daily laxative.
    3. Swallow the medication without gulping air.
    4. Maintain adequate fiber in the diet.
    5. Take the medication with a noncarbonated beverage.

Drugs Used to Treat Hypertension

Answer Key: Textbook page references are provided as a guide for answering these questions. A complete answer key is provided to your instructor.

MATCHING

Match the term on the right with the definition on the left.

Definition

1. _____ a disease characterized by an elevation of the blood pressure

2. _____ the most common form of hypertension

3. _____ drugs that bind to angiotensin II receptor sites

4. _____ the difference between the systolic and diastolic pressure

5. _____ drugs that cause volume depletion, sodium excretion, and vasodilation of peripheral arterioles

6. _____ the pressure in the blood vessels when the heart muscle relaxes between contractions

7. _____ drugs that cause arteriolar smooth muscle relaxation

8. _____ high blood pressure that occurs after the development of another disorder

9. _____ drugs that inhibit angiotensin I converting enzyme

10. _____ drugs that inhibit cardiac response to sympathetic nerve stimulation by blocking beta receptors

11. _____ the pressure with which the blood is pumped from the heart

12. _____ drugs that inhibit the movement of calcium ions across a cell membrane

13. _____ this accounts for 90% of all clinical cases of high blood pressure, cause unknown

14. _____ this is determined by the stroke volume, heart rate, and venous capacitance

15. _____ the average pressure throughout each cycle of the heartbeat

Term

a. secondary hypertension
b. pulse pressure
c. systolic blood pressure
d. mean arterial pressure
e. diastolic blood pressure
f. hypertension
g. beta-adrenergic blockers
h. cardiac output
i. primary hypertension
j. systolic hypertension
k. diuretic
l. ACE inhibitors
m. angiotensin II receptor blockers
n. calcium channel blockers
o. direct vasodilators

REVIEW QUESTIONS

Scenario: A 42-year-old man came into the clinic complaining of frequent headaches and was diagnosed with stage 1 hypertension. He was referred to the education specialist for further instructions on lifestyle modification and initiation of drug therapy.

Differentiate between primary and secondary hypertension.

16. A patient has a blood pressure reading of 138/85 mm Hg. The nurse identifies this patient as having which classification of hypertension? *(342)*
    1. Normal
    2. Stage 1
    3. Stage 2
    4. Elevated

17. A nurse was discussing the difference between primary and secondary hypertension with the patient in the scenario. Which response by the nurse would be appropriate? *(341)*
    1. "Primary hypertension is curable, while secondary hypertension is only controllable."
    2. "There is no difference between primary and secondary hypertension; both of them can be cured."
    3. "Primary hypertension occurs during adolescence, while secondary hypertension happens to people after they reach adulthood."
    4. "Primary hypertension occurs about 90% of the time and has no known cause, while secondary hypertension occurs after the development of another disorder."

18. Which conditions are identifiable causes of hypertension? *(Select all that apply.)* *(341)*
    1. Sleep apnea
    2. Chronic kidney disease
    3. Primary aldosteronism
    4. Marfan's syndrome
    5. Thyroid disease

19. Various types of antihypertensive agents have an effect on which system that plays an important role in the development of hypertension? *(351)*
    1. RAAS cascade
    2. CIWA scale
    3. Coagulation cascade
    4. Adrenergic blocking system

Summarize nursing assessments and interventions used for the treatment of hypertension.

20. What will the nurse do to measure a patient's blood pressure? *(Select all that apply.)* *(348)*
    1. Use an appropriately sized cuff.
    2. Verify reading in the opposite arm.
    3. Support the arm at the same level as the heart.
    4. Sit the patient in a chair with feet dangling off the floor.
    5. Inflate the cuff 50 mm Hg above the point at which the radial pulse disappears.

21. Which drug class includes the most commonly prescribed antihypertensive agents? *(350)*
    1. Diuretics
    2. ACE inhibitors
    3. Angiotensin II receptor blockers
    4. Calcium channel blockers

22. For patients who are diagnosed with hypertension, further evaluation must be obtained to determine what? *(Select all that apply.)* *(341)*
    1. Identify possible causes of hypertension
    2. Any history of tonsillectomy or appendectomy
    3. Any presence of target organ damage
    4. Current understanding of the drugs used for hypertension
    5. Laboratory tests to identify any cardiovascular disease

23. Systolic blood pressure is the pressure exerted by the heart as blood is pumped out; diastolic blood pressure is the pressure present when? *(340)*
    1. During the peak of physical activity
    2. After the blood returns to the heart
    3. After the valves of the heart close
    4. During the resting phase of the heartbeat

24. The nurse needs to educate the patient in the scenario regarding what in the medication regimen? *(Select all that apply.)* *(349)*
    1. Dosage
    2. Time and frequency
    3. Adverse effects to watch for
    4. The need for daily weights
    5. How often to perform toe wiggles and rising on the toes

25. The purpose of controlling hypertension is to reduce the frequency of which disorders? *(Select all that apply.)* *(342)*
    1. Stroke
    2. Renal failure
    3. Hyperthyroidism
    4. Heart failure
    5. Bladder cancer

Identify recommended lifestyle modifications after a diagnosis of hypertension.

26. When discussing the modifications that are recommended for the patient in the scenario, the nurse will review which factors? *(Select all that apply.)* *(349)*
    1. Weight reduction
    2. Using the DASH diet
    3. Stress management training
    4. Maintaining usual sodium intake
    5. Increase physical activity to moderate exercise

27. What are some lifestyle modifications for the treatment of hypertension? *(Select all that apply.)* *(349)*
    1. Eating more fruits and vegetables
    2. Consuming more dairy products per day
    3. Reducing the amount of dietary sodium intake
    4. Limiting consumption of alcohol to no more than two drinks per day
    5. Increasing physical activity to 40 minutes, three or four times per week

28. A patient asks the nurse how much exercise is considered enough for the control of blood pressure. The nurse knows that a range of 4-9 mm Hg of approximate systolic pressure reduction can occur with engaging in regular physical activity how often? *(343)*
    1. For as little as 3 days a week
    2. For at least 40 minutes per session
    3. For 15-20 minutes a week at the most
    4. For as little as 90 minutes a week

29. The nurse was instructing the patient in the scenario regarding lifestyle modification and recognized that further education was needed after the patient made which statement? *(342)*
    1. "So my plan is to start losing weight gradually so I can keep it off."
    2. "I know that I will have to stop eating tortilla chips since they have a lot of salt."
    3. "I understand that I need to walk more than just twice a week, so I think I will walk four times a week."
    4. "Since I will be started on drug therapy for my high blood pressure, I do not need to change my habits."

Identify initial options and progression of medicines used to treat hypertension.

30. The nurse expects that the patient in the scenario may be started on which drug class? *(Select all that apply.)* *(343)*
    1. Diuretics
    2. Beta blockers
    3. Calcium channel blockers
    4. Aldosterone receptor antagonists
    5. Angiotensin-converting enzyme inhibitors

31. After being on a thiazide for several months, a patient being treated for stage 1 hypertension will most likely have which medication added because the target blood pressure was not attained? *(344)*
    1. aliskiren (Tekturna)
    2. eplerenone (Inspra)
    3. nifedipine (Procardia)
    4. spironolactone (Aldactone)

32. For patients who have stage 2 hypertension and need to be started on two-drug combinations for blood pressure control, which drug classes may be started? *(Select all that apply.)* *(353, 355)*
    1. Diuretics
    2. Renin inhibitors
    3. Angiotensin II receptor blockers
    4. Calcium channel blockers
    5. Angiotensin-converting enzyme inhibitors

33. The patient in the scenario asks the nurse about risk factors for developing hypertension and the nurse's response includes which statement? *(Select all that apply.)* *(341)*
    1. "The risk factors that cannot be managed are your age, gender, and race."
    2. "The best way to treat high blood pressure is to limit your salt intake."
    3. "With exercise and proper diet, you can start to help manage your blood pressure."
    4. "Lifestyle changes are important to recognize as part of the management of hypertension."
    5. "You will need to get a low-stress job since that is the best way to manage your high blood pressure."

34. While discussing the best way to change diet habits with a patient who has hypertension, the nurse asks the patient about what? *(346)*
    1. To estimate the percentage of total daily calories from fats
    2. To restrict the amount of dairy products in the diet
    3. The portion size and number of servings the patient eats of refined carbohydrates and sodium
    4. How foods are prepared in the home and if fried foods are preferred over baked or broiled

35. A patient in the scenario was discussing how to manage his blood pressure with the nurse and mentioned that he likes to smoke an occasional cigar. What is the best response from the nurse? *(345)*
    1. "How often would you say is 'occasional'?"
    2. "That should be okay; smoking does not affect your blood pressure."
    3. "You will need to stop smoking altogether, since that is very bad for you."
    4. "Did you know that smoking will cause the diuretic you are on to be ineffective?"

Identify and summarize the action of five drug classes used to treat hypertension.

36. Which drugs are the direct vasodilators? *(Select all that apply.)* *(365-366)*
    1. methyldopa
    2. nitroprusside sodium (Nitropress)
    3. guanfacine (Tenex)
    4. hydralazine
    5. aliskiren (Tekturna)

37. Which class of antihypertensive agents lowers blood pressure by blocking a very potent vasoconstrictor from binding to the receptor sites in vascular smooth muscle, brain, heart, kidneys, and adrenal glands? *(355)*
    1. Beta blockers
    2. Angiotensin II receptor blockers
    3. Calcium channel blockers
    4. Aldosterone receptor antagonists

38. If patients develop a chronic, dry, nonproductive cough and are taking which antihypertensive agent, they will need to contact their healthcare provider to get a different agent? *(352-353)*
    1. metoprolol
    2. hydralazine
    3. captopril
    4. amlodipine

39. Calcium channel blockers are used for the reduction of blood pressure and have what other effect? *(Select all that apply.)* *(359-360)*
    1. Reduce the afterload of the heart
    2. Peripheral vasodilating effects
    3. Increase the sodium excretion in the kidneys
    4. Increase the preload of the heart
    5. Peripheral vasoconstricting effects

40. The drug prazosin, an alpha-1 adrenergic blocking agent, has which therapeutic effects? *(Select all that apply.)* *(360, 362)*
    1. Improving memory
    2. Reducing blood lipids
    3. Improving urine flow
    4. Reducing blood pressure
    5. Reducing gastric acid production

Drugs Used to Treat Dysrhythmias

Answer Key: Textbook page references are provided as a guide for answering these questions. A complete answer key is provided to your instructor.

MATCHING

Match the term on the right with the definition on the left.

Definition

1. _____ an obstruction of conduction pathways, resulting in delayed conduction
2. _____ a disturbance in the normal electrical conduction of the heart, resulting in abnormal heart muscle contraction
3. _____ ringing in the ears
4. _____ digoxin
5. _____ a type of supraventricular dysrhythmia
6. _____ the electrical system of the heart
7. _____ the pacemaker cells in the conduction system
8. _____ dyspnea, chest pain, fatigue, edema, syncope, and palpitations

Term

a. conduction system
b. this antidysrhythmic agent works by slowing the conduction through the AV node
c. dysrhythmia
d. atrioventricular blocks
e. SA node
f. six cardinal signs of cardiovascular disease
g. paroxysmal supraventricular tachycardia (PSVT)
h. tinnitus

REVIEW QUESTIONS

Scenario: An 89-year-old male patient was admitted to the hospital after falling and fracturing his arm. He has a history of atrial fibrillation and had a permanent pacemaker implanted several years ago.

Describe the anatomic structures and conduction system of the heart.

9. The conduction system of the heart begins in the pacemaker cells known as what? *(368)*
   1. Purkinje fibers
   2. Bundle of His
   3. Sinoatrial (SA) node
   4. Atrioventricular (AV) node
10. Identify the sequence of the electrical current as it travels through the conduction system of the heart in the correct order. *(368)*
    1. _____ Purkinje fibers
    2. _____ AV node
    3. _____ Bundle of His
    4. _____ SA node

11. When the electrical current passes through the SA node, it causes what to happen? *(368)*
    1. The ventricles to contract
    2. The heart muscle to contract from the apex
    3. The atrial muscle to contract and fill the ventricles
    4. The blood to be pumped out through the aorta
12. Dysrhythmias may be caused by abnormal pacemaker cells, as well as what other cause? *(368)*
    1. An opening in the Purkinje fibers
    2. A contraction of the atrial muscle
    3. The flow of blood through the SA node
    4. A blockage of the normal electrical pathways
13. Dysrhythmias that develop above the bundle of His are called *supraventricular dysrhythmias*, and include which ones? *(Select all that apply.) (369)*
    1. Sinus bradycardia
    2. Normal sinus rhythm
    3. Atrial flutter / atrial fibrillation
    4. Premature atrial contractions
    5. Paroxysmal supraventricular tachycardia

14. Dysrhythmias that develop below the bundle of His are referred to as *ventricular dysrhythmias* and include which ones? *(Select all that apply.) (369)*
    1. Sinus tachycardia
    2. Atrial tachycardia
    3. Ventricular fibrillation
    4. Ventricular tachycardia
    5. Premature ventricular contractions

Identify the classification of drugs used to treat dysrhythmias.

15. The goal of treatment for dysrhythmias is to restore normal sinus rhythm and what else? *(369)*
    1. To speed up the rate of the heart
    2. To increase the contractility of the heart muscle
    3. To improve the output from the atrial muscle
    4. To prevent recurrence of life-threatening dysrhythmias

16. Of the medications that the patient in the scenario is taking, the nurse recognizes which medication for the treatment of atrial fibrillation? *(370)*
    1. irbesartan (Avapro)
    2. tramadol (Ultram)
    3. omeprazole (Prilosec)
    4. digoxin (Lanoxin)

17. Which class of antidysrhythmics acts as myocardial depressants by inhibiting sodium ion movement in the heart? *(369)*
    1. Class I agents
    2. Class II agents
    3. Class III agents
    4. Class IV agents

18. Which class of antidysrhythmic drugs is effective in inhibiting cardiac response to sympathetic nerve stimulation, and as a result, reduces heart rate, blood pressure, and cardiac output? *(375)*
    1. Calcium channel blockers
    2. Beta-adrenergic blockers
    3. Potassium channel blockers
    4. Sodium channel blockers

Identify baseline nursing assessments that should be implemented during the treatment of dysrhythmias.

19. Which methods are used to assess dysrhythmias that patients develop? *(Select all that apply.) (370)*
    1. Laboratory values
    2. Electric shock therapy
    3. Exercise electrocardiography
    4. Electrocardiogram (ECG) monitoring
    5. Electrophysiologic studies (EPS)

20. The nurse recognizes that it is important to monitor the hourly urine output in a patient with dysrhythmias because this may indicate what? *(371)*
    1. The function of the atrial muscle
    2. The patient's cardiac output
    3. Whether the kidneys are being adequately perfused
    4. Whether the peripheral tissues are being adequately perfused

21. Assessing a cardiac patient for level of consciousness is one of the important baseline assessments that the nurse will perform to determine adequate: *(371)*
    1. peripheral perfusion.
    2. cerebral tissue perfusion.
    3. renal perfusion.
    4. lung perfusion.

Cite common adverse effects that may be observed with the administration of antidysrhythmic drugs.

22. When given intravenously, amiodarone needs to be administered how? *(376)*
    1. Slowly over an hour, and flushed immediately
    2. Slowly over an hour, then followed with a continuous drip
    3. Quickly over 10 minutes, then flushed immediately
    4. Quickly over 10 minutes, then followed with a continuous drip

23. The nurse needs to monitor which vital signs of patients who are taking antidysrhythmic drugs? *(Select all that apply.) (371)*
    1. Respirations
    2. Pulse quality
    3. Oxygen saturation
    4. Adequate intake
    5. Blood pressure in both arms

24. The laboratory tests that should be monitored for patients taking antidysrhythmic drugs include which values? *(Select all that apply.) (371)*
    1. Gastric pH
    2. Electrolytes
    3. Thyroid levels
    4. Arterial blood gases
    5. Creatine kinase (CK-MB)

25. Amiodarone may cause serious adverse effects, and the patient will need periodic tests to determine any effect on which function(s)? *(Select all that apply.) (376)*
    1. Hearing loss
    2. Thyroid function
    3. Liver function
    4. Visual disturbance
    5. Pulmonary function

26. The nurse is teaching the patient in the scenario that he will be started on propafenone (Rythmol) for further control of his atrial fibrillation. The nurse teaches him to be alert for which common adverse effects of the drug? *(Select all that apply.) (375)*
    1. Tremors
    2. Dizziness
    3. Constipation
    4. Nausea and vomiting
    5. Sleep disturbances

27. Caution must be taken with patients who receive a neuromuscular blockade while also receiving quinidine because of what effect? *(373)*
    1. Quinidine will increase bleeding time.
    2. CNS response to quinidine causes lethargy.
    3. Respiratory muscles are stimulated with quinidine.
    4. Quinidine may prolong the effects of these muscle relaxants.
28. When assessing the patient who is taking quinidine, following the administration of succinylcholine for a biopsy, the nurse observes for which signs? *(373)*
    1. Tinnitus
    2. Respiratory depression
    3. Bleeding gums and bruises
    4. Anorexia, nausea, and vomiting

List the six cardinal signs of cardiovascular disease.
29. Which is the cardinal sign of cardiovascular disease that involves the respiratory system? *(370-371)*
    1. Dyspnea
    2. Palpitations
    3. Edema
    4. Syncope

30. The patient in the scenario began to feel tired easily and starting to take naps in the afternoon. Which sign of cardiovascular disease does this represent? *(370-371)*
    1. Chest pain
    2. Fatigue
    3. Edema
    4. Syncope
31. When monitoring patients for signs of cardiovascular disease, the nurse will observe for edema. Where are the specific areas of the body most likely to show signs of edema? *(Select all that apply.)* *(371)*
    1. Arms
    2. Mid-calf
    3. Ankles
    4. Thigh
    5. Hands
32. The patient in the scenario told the nurse that he felt as though his heart was skipping some beats. The nurse recognized this symptom as which one of the six cardinal signs of cardiovascular disease? *(371)*
    1. Dyspnea
    2. Syncope
    3. Fatigue
    4. Palpitations

Drugs Used to Treat Angina Pectoris

Answer Key: Textbook page references are provided as a guide for answering these questions. A complete answer key is provided to your instructor.

MATCHING
Match the term on the right with the definition on the left.

Definition

1. _____ occurs while the patient is at rest, caused by vasospasms of the coronary artery, diagnosed by combination of history and exercise testing

2. _____ precipitated by physical exertion or stress, lasts only a few minutes, relieved by nitroglycerin

3. _____ unpredictable chest pain; changes in onset, frequency, duration, and intensity

4. _____ supply of oxygen needed by the heart cells is inadequate

5. _____ feeling of chest discomfort arising from the heart

Term

a. unstable angina
b. ischemia
c. chronic stable angina
d. angina pectoris
e. variant angina

REVIEW QUESTIONS

Scenario: A 52-year-old male patient was admitted through the emergency department to a telemetry unit after experiencing sudden substernal chest pain radiating down his left arm, feeling faint, and indigestion. He was a history of urinary retention, palpitations, insomnia, and depression.

Define angina pectoris and identify assessment data needed to evaluate an anginal attack.

6. The underlying cause of anginal pain is a result of what? *(382)*
   1. A cardiac dysrhythmia
   2. A severe increase in blood pressure
   3. Decreased circulation to the chest muscles
   4. The lack of an adequate oxygen supply to the cells in the heart

7. The patient in the scenario has various presenting symptoms of angina (in addition to the substernal chest pain radiating down his left arm), which include what? *(Select all that apply.)* *(382)*
   1. Palpitations
   2. Depression
   3. Insomnia
   4. Feeling faint
   5. Urinary retention

8. The nurse needs to gather which assessment data from patients who present with angina? *(Select all that apply.)* *(383-385)*
   1. Any smoking history
   2. What medications are being taken
   3. Vital signs and pulse checks
   4. The onset, duration, and intensity of pain
   5. The degree of understanding regarding lifestyle modifications

Differentiate between chronic stable angina and unstable angina and the drug therapy used for each type.

9. The patient in the scenario is considered to have which type of angina? *(382)*
   1. Variant angina
   2. Unstable angina
   3. Chronic angina
   4. Stable angina

10. What is the difference between unstable angina and chronic stable angina? *(382)*
    1. Chronic angina is relieved with rest and unstable angina is relieved with exercise.
    2. Unstable angina is caused by vasospasm and chronic angina is caused by a fixed obstruction.
    3. Chronic angina is unpredictable in nature and unstable angina occurs at regular intervals.
    4. Unstable angina is relieved with nitroglycerin and chronic angina is relieved with statin drugs.
11. The nurse explaining to the patient in the scenario the treatment goals for angina will include which statement(s) in the discussion? *(Select all that apply.)* *(382)*
    1. "The choices you have for treatment therapies are designed to prevent a heart attack."
    2. "Your healthcare team wants to improve quality of life by relieving your anginal pain."
    3. "You may have the choice of either angioplasty or bypass surgery depending on the results of further tests."
    4. "Depending on the results of your tests, you will be instructed to make changes in your lifestyle prior to starting on any drug therapy."
    5. "In the future, when you have anginal pain, you can take a Tylenol first before taking any nitroglycerin."
12. What is included in premedication assessments that the nurse should perform prior to administering nitrates for patients with heart disease? *(Select all that apply.)* *(386)*
    1. Any history of gastritis
    2. The location, duration, and pattern of pain
    3. When the most recent nitrate was used
    4. Checking laboratory results of HDLs
    5. The ability to place the medication under the tongue correctly

Describe the actions of nitrates, beta-adrenergic blockers, calcium channel blockers, and angiotensin-converting enzyme inhibitors on the myocardial tissue of the heart.

13. The desired action of calcium channel blockers in the treatment of angina is to have what effect? *(Select all that apply.)* *(389)*
    1. Decrease the workload of the heart
    2. Decrease resistance to blood flow
    3. Decrease the peripheral circulation
    4. Dilate the peripheral blood vessels
    5. Increase myocardial blood supply via coronary arteries
14. The common adverse effects associated with angiotensin-converting enzyme inhibitors include: *(Select all that apply.)* *(390)*
    1. fainting.
    2. tachycardia.
    3. nasal congestion.
    4. hypotension with dizziness.
    5. indigestion or heartburn.

15. Patients with a history of which disorder are at the highest risk for complications associated with use of beta-adrenergic blockers for the treatment of angina? *(389)*
    1. Anemia
    2. Gastric ulcer
    3. Respiratory disorders
    4. High blood pressure
16. Nitrates are used for therapy to treat angina because they have which effect? *(385)*
    1. Nitrates increase the serum creatinine.
    2. Nitrates prevent platelet aggregation.
    3. Nitrates lower the amount of circulating LDLs.
    4. Nitrates cause blood vessels to dilate, allowing more blood flow.
17. ACE inhibitors are effective in relieving anginal attacks because they have which effect? *(390)*
    1. ACE inhibitors prolong the QT interval.
    2. ACE inhibitors decrease serum creatinine.
    3. ACE inhibitors lower the amount of circulating LDLs.
    4. ACE inhibitors promote vasodilation and minimize platelet aggregation.
18. Calcium channel blockers are used to relieve anginal attacks because they have which effect? *(389)*
    1. Calcium channel blockers prevent platelet aggregation.
    2. Calcium channel blockers lower the amount of circulating LDLs.
    3. Calcium channel blockers increase calcium levels in the blood.
    4. Calcium channel blockers dilate the peripheral vessels and inhibit smooth muscle contractions.
19. Common adverse effects of nitrate therapy may include which symptoms? *(Select all that apply.)* *(388)*
    1. Nausea
    2. Tolerance
    3. Bradycardia
    4. Excessive hypotension
    5. Prolonged headache
20. The nurse includes which statements when teaching a patient about the use of nitroglycerin spray (Nitrolingual)? *(Select all that apply.)* *(386)*
    1. "Do not inhale or swallow the spray."
    2. "Spray the dose onto the roof of your mouth."
    3. "Do not shake the container before administration."
    4. "Hold the canister vertically when administering the medication."
    5. "Call 911 if chest pain is not relieved by one dose within 5 minutes."

Identify risk factor management and healthy lifestyle changes that are taught to prevent disease progression and myocardial infarction or death.

21. The nurse will teach a patient to do what at the first sign of an anginal attack? *(386)*
    1. Call 911.
    2. Sit or lie down.
    3. Take two nitroglycerin tablets.
    4. Take an extra dose of transdermal nitroglycerin.
22. In addition to weight control and a structured exercise program, the nurse should also educate the patient on other ways of improving cardiovascular health such as managing which conditions? *(Select all that apply.)* *(383)*
    1. Migraines
    2. Dyslipidemia
    3. Hypertension
    4. Hypothyroidism
    5. Diabetes mellitus
23. The nurse was explaining to the patient in the scenario about the need to avoid activities that precipitate attacks of angina, which may include: *(Select all that apply.)* *(382)*
    1. watching TV.
    2. eating a light lunch.
    3. lifting heavy boxes.
    4. climbing a flight of stairs.
    5. exposure to cold temperatures.

Drugs Used to Treat Peripheral Vascular Disease

chapter

25

Answer Key: Textbook page references are provided as a guide for answering these questions. A complete answer key is provided to your instructor.

MATCHING

Match the term on the right with the definition on the left.

Definition

1. _____ a condition caused by vasospasms of the blood vessels triggered by unknown mechanisms

2. _____ numbness with a tingling sensation

3. _____ vasoconstriction of blood vessels

4. _____ pain secondary to lack of oxygen to the muscles during exercise

5. _____ obstructive arterial disease resulting from atherosclerotic plaque formation

Term

a. arteriosclerosis obliterans
b. intermittent claudication
c. paresthesias
d. Raynaud's disease
e. vasospasm

REVIEW QUESTIONS

Scenario: An 81-year-old male patient was admitted to the hospital with complaints of progressive pain in both legs with activity that no longer goes away when the activity is stopped.

Describe the baseline assessments needed to evaluate a patient with peripheral vascular disease.

6. The nurse needs to assess for what after patients are started on vasodilating agents? *(397)*
   1. Paresthesias
   2. Pulsus paradoxus
   3. Orthostatic hypotension
   4. Thrombus formation

7. What is the most common form of peripheral vascular disease? *(393)*
   1. Arteritis
   2. Arteriosclerosis obliterans
   3. Raynaud's disease
   4. Coarctation of the aorta

8. Baseline assessments the nurse will gather on the patient in the scenario regarding peripheral vascular disease include which factors? *(Select all that apply.)* *(395)*
   1. Limb pain
   2. Skin temperature
   3. Respiratory rate
   4. Peripheral pulses
   5. Presence of edema

9. The patient in the scenario has symptoms that may indicate intermittent claudication that is progressing. The nurse would expect which findings as further evidence of arteriosclerosis? *(Select all that apply.)* *(393)*
   1. Paresthesias
   2. Pink-colored skin
   3. Poor pulses in the feet
   4. Warmer skin temperature of the legs
   5. Cooler skin temperature of the legs

10. The phrase *peripheral vascular disease* can be applied to a variety of disorders and illnesses such as what? *(Select all that apply.)* *(393)*
    1. Aortic stenosis
    2. Arterial spasms
    3. Coronary heart disease
    4. Arterial disease affecting the extremities.
    5. Venous obstructions caused by thrombosis

Identify specific measures that the patient can use to improve peripheral circulation and prevent the complications of peripheral vascular disease.

11. What do physical findings on the lower extremities associated with peripheral vascular disease include? *(Select all that apply.)* *(393)*
    1. Edema
    2. Numbness to sensation
    3. Waxy, pale, and dry skin
    4. Reduced arterial pulsations on palpation
    5. Warmer temperature of the skin of the extremity

12. Without specific orders to do so from the healthcare provider, patients with peripheral vascular disease should be taught not to elevate their extremities above the level of what organ? *(396)*
    1. The bladder
    2. The heart
    3. The liver
    4. The eyes

13. What are the most cost-effective and successful forms of treatment for peripheral vascular disease? *(Select all that apply.)* *(396)*
    1. Exercise
    2. Medications
    3. Weight reduction
    4. Smoking cessation
    5. Dietary modification

Identify the systemic effects to expect when peripheral vasodilating agents are administered.

14. The nurse teaching self-assessment to the patient in the scenario advises which measures to promote tissue perfusion? *(Select all that apply.)* *(395)*
    1. Reduce and stop smoking.
    2. Wear constricting stockings.
    3. Elevate the head of the bed.
    4. Elevate the extremities when sitting.
    5. Visually inspect the feet to note any skin breakdown.

15. Which agent used for treatment of intermittent claudication is thought to work by increasing erythrocyte flexibility? *(397)*
    1. verapamil (Calan)
    2. pentoxifylline
    3. adenosine (Adenocard)
    4. cilostazol

16. Which classes of drugs have been used successfully for the treatment of Raynaud's disease? *(Select all that apply.)* *(394)*
    1. Direct vasodilators
    2. Calcium channel blockers
    3. Adrenergic antagonists
    4. Sodium channel blockers
    5. Angiotensin-converting enzyme inhibitors

17. The nurse collecting assessment data on the patient in the scenario for evidence of circulatory impairment in his legs needs to include which findings? *(Select all that apply.)* *(395)*
    1. Check the pedal and radial pulses.
    2. Compare the pulses in the extremities.
    3. Ask about the frequency and volume of alcoholic beverages consumed.
    4. Determine the number of cigarettes or cigars smoked daily.
    5. Use a Doppler ultrasound to help determine peripheral blood flow.

Explain why hypotension and tachycardia occur frequently with the use of pentoxifylline and cilostazol.

18. Nitroglycerin ointment was used as a treatment for Raynaud's disease, but which adverse effects limit its use? *(Select all that apply.)* *(394)*
    1. Dizziness
    2. Headache
    3. Numbness and tingling of hands
    4. Postural hypotension
    5. Intermittent claudication

19. Because certain medications used for the treatment of peripheral vascular disease cause vasodilation, the nurse will need to instruct the patient to do what to prevent side effects? *(394)*
    1. Rise slowly.
    2. Cross their legs when sitting.
    3. Drink four glasses of water daily.
    4. Encourage a diet high in salt intake.

20. Instructions for an individual with peripheral vascular disease should include which recommendation? *(Select all that apply.)* *(396)*
    1. Reduce or totally quit smoking.
    2. Elevate the extremities above the heart.
    3. Use self-care measures to promote peripheral circulation.
    4. Avoid standing or sitting for prolonged periods of time.
    5. Encourage patient to wear tight-fitting anklets or socks.

21. The nurse will include which statement when teaching a patient about pentoxifylline (Trental) for treatment of peripheral vascular disease? *(398)*
    1. "This drug should be taken 30 minutes before or 2 hours after eating."
    2. "This drug may cause your blood pressure to be lower."
    3. "If this drug makes you feel dizzy, stop taking it immediately."
    4. "You will need to have a blood test called an INR to monitor the effects of this drug."

22. What direct vasodilator is used for the treatment of Raynaud's disease? *(394)*
    1. hydralazine
    2. nitroprusside
    3. nitroglycerin ointment
    4. nitroglycerin sublingual

Cite both pharmacologic and nonpharmacologic goals of the treatment for peripheral vascular disease.

23. The nurse was discussing with the patient some of the options that the healthcare provider and patient had reviewed earlier in the day. To clarify the patient's options, the nurse could make which therapeutic statement? *(394)*
    1. "The provider talked to you about surgical options when you feel the medications are no longer effective."
    2. "The surgical options are the way to go and get this problem taken care of, in my opinion."
    3. "The provider said to you that amputation of your leg is the next step, rather than angioplasty or bypass grafting."
    4. "There is nothing further we can do for you. You will just have to suffer because there are no more options available to you other than the medications."

24. Which two agents are the only ones approved by the FDA for treatment of intermittent claudication caused by occlusive arterial disease? *(394)*
    1. clopidogrel and vorapaxar
    2. verapamil and nifedipine
    3. pentoxifylline and cilostazol
    4. papaverine and isoxsuprine

25. A patient asks the nurse what can be done to decrease the occurrence and severity of vasospastic attacks of Raynaud's disease. How does the nurse respond? *(Select all that apply.)* *(394)*
    1. "Most attacks of Raynaud's disease can be stopped by avoiding hot temperatures."
    2. "Tobacco use is highly associated with vasospastic attacks of Raynaud's disease."
    3. "It is not known what really triggers the vasospastic attacks seen with Raynaud's disease."
    4. "The signs and symptoms associated with Raynaud's disease are due to vasospasm of the arteries of the skin of the hands, fingers, and sometimes toes."
    5. "Most people have Raynaud's disease for a few years and then it goes away."

Drugs Used to Treat Thromboembolic Disorders

chapter
26

Answer Key: Textbook page references are provided as a guide for answering these questions. A complete answer key is provided to your instructor.

MATCHING

Match the term on the right with the definition on the left.

Definition

1. _____ drug class that inhibits platelet aggregation

2. _____ drug class that is active against factor Xa and thrombin

3. _____ triggered by sources outside the blood vessels, such as tissue extract or thromboplastin

4. _____ drug class that inhibits thrombin, preventing the conversion of fibrinogen to fibrin

5. _____ drug class that acts by blocking receptors on platelets, preventing clot formation

6. _____ a small fragment of a thrombus that breaks off

7. _____ drug class that causes the dissolution of fibrin clots

8. _____ a fibrin blood clot

9. _____ activated when a blood vessel is injured and collagen in the vessel wall is exposed

Term

a. thrombus
b. embolus
c. intrinsic clotting pathway
d. extrinsic clotting pathway
e. fibrinolytic agents
f. platelet inhibitors
g. anticoagulants
h. thrombin inhibitors
i. glycoprotein IIb/IIIa inhibitors

REVIEW QUESTIONS

Scenario: An 82-year-old woman who was admitted to the hospital with a stroke has a history of atrial fibrillation and noncompliance with medications.

Explain the primary purposes of anticoagulant therapy.

10. What are major causes of thrombus formation? *(Select all that apply.)* *(401)*
    1. Anemia
    2. Claudication
    3. Heart failure
    4. Surgery and the postoperative period
    5. Immobility with venous stasis

11. Which factors trigger blood clot formation? *(Select all that apply.)* *(401)*
    1. Circulating clotting proteins
    2. Increased blood viscosity
    3. Damage to a blood vessel wall
    4. Fibrinogen activated by thrombin to soluble fibrin
    5. The presence of potassium in the cells

12. What is the effect on the blood clot when patients are placed on anticoagulants? *(403)*
    1. It will be dissolved
    2. It is prevented from growing
    3. It becomes trapped in a capillary
    4. It will circulate throughout the bloodstream

13. What is the difference between red and white blood clots? *(402)*
    1. Red clots are fragile and break easily; white clots are stationary.
    2. Red clots develop in arteries; white clots develop in veins.
    3. Red clots are made up of platelets and fibrin; white clots are made of fibrin and erythrocytes.
    4. Red clots are made up of fibrin and erythrocytes; white clots are made of platelets and fibrin.

14. What routine laboratory tests are run to assess the clotting process and ensure that occult bleeding is not present? *(Select all that apply.)* *(402)*
    1. Stool guaiac test
    2. Prothrombin time (PT)
    3. Activated clotting time (ACT)
    4. Renin angiotensin aldosterone
    5. International Normalized Ratio (INR)

Describe conditions that place an individual at risk for developing blood clots and nursing interventions used to prevent these conditions.

15. Which conditions put patients at risk for developing blood clots? *(Select all that apply.)* *(401)*
    1. Heart failure
    2. Certain types of cancers
    3. Pregnancy and oral contraceptives
    4. Immobilization or trauma of the lower limbs
    5. Eating large amounts of green leafy vegetables

16. The patient in the scenario is at risk for developing a clot that breaks off and creates a pulmonary embolism because of what factors? *(Select all that apply.)* *(403)*
    1. The patient is noncompliant with her medications.
    2. She is taking her medications on a regular basis.
    3. She has atrial fibrillation, which is known to cause blood clots.
    4. She walks slowly because of her advanced age and it slows her blood flow.
    5. The healthcare provider had not prescribed the correct medications to prevent a blood clot.

17. What nursing actions can help prevent the formation of a clot in those patients who are at risk for developing blood clots? *(Select all that apply.)* *(403-404)*
    1. Restrict fluid intake to 1 liter/day.
    2. Assess perfusion of extremities.
    3. Flex the patient's knees when on bedrest.
    4. Review laboratory data such as hematocrit and platelet count.
    5. Apply sequential compression devices as prescribed by the healthcare provider.

18. The nurse knows which types of patients are at risk for developing clots? *(Select all that apply.)* *(403)*
    1. Patients who are on prolonged bedrest
    2. Patients who have had a history of blood clots
    3. Patients who limit their intake of green leafy vegetables
    4. Patients who have recently had orthopedic or thoracic surgery
    5. Patient who are adequately controlled on anticoagulation therapy

Identify the actions of platelet inhibitors, anticoagulants, thrombin inhibitors, and fibrinolytic agents.

19. What is the primary purpose of anticoagulants when administered after a blood clot is discovered? *(403)*
    1. Dissolve the existing clot.
    2. Prevent the clot from forming.
    3. Decrease the size of the clot.
    4. Prevent the extension of the existing clot.

20. When a small fragment of a thrombus breaks off and circulates until it becomes trapped causing a cerebral embolism, the treatment of choice would be to use what class of drug? *(403)*
    1. Anticoagulant
    2. Thrombin inhibitor
    3. Platelet inhibitor
    4. Fibrinolytic agent

21. Platelet inhibitors are used to prevent clot formation in which conditions? *(Select all that apply.)* *(405)*
    1. Mitral stenosis
    2. Strokes (CVAs)
    3. Thrombocytopenia
    4. Myocardial infarction
    5. Transient ischemic attacks (TIAs)

22. When patients are receiving anticoagulant therapy, the nurse should instruct them on which measures to prevent clot formation? *(Select all that apply.)* *(404)*
    1. Regular ambulation
    2. Not to flex the knees
    3. Active or passive leg exercises
    4. Placing pressure against the popliteal space behind the knees
    5. Standing or sitting motionless for prolonged periods of time

23. Which adverse effects need to be reported when patients are taking apixaban (Eliquis)? *(Select all that apply.)* *(409)*
    1. Ataxia
    2. Nystagmus
    3. Hematuria
    4. Easy bruising
    5. Black tarry stools

24. The therapeutic effect of heparin is monitored by which laboratory tests? *(Select all that apply.)* *(414)*
    1. Protime
    2. Platelets
    3. aPTT
    4. Anti-factor Xa
    5. Hematocrit

25. The thrombin inhibitor dabigatran (Pradaxa) has which major advantage over anticoagulants used for reducing the risk of stroke or systemic embolism? **(417)**
    1. When metabolized, it takes the form of four active metabolites.
    2. The capsules are taken two times daily with or without food.
    3. The drug does not require monitoring of blood tests to adjust the dosage.
    4. Baseline blood pressure readings need to be obtained supine and standing.

Describe specific monitoring procedures and laboratory data used to detect hemorrhage in the patient taking anticoagulants.

26. Which premedication assessments should be performed by the nurse before administering aspirin as a platelet inhibitor? *(Select all that apply.)* **(405)**
    1. Serum potassium levels
    2. Neurologic assessment
    3. Gastrointestinal symptoms
    4. Concurrent use of antihypertensives
    5. Baseline serum glucose if on oral hypoglycemic

27. The nurse will observe for which specific events to detect for internal bleeding in patients on IV heparin? *(Select all that apply.)* **(414)**
    1. Paresthesias
    2. Increasing pulse
    3. Cold, clammy skin
    4. Decreasing blood pressure
    5. Disoriented sensorium

28. Nurses will educate patients on what to report when on Coumadin therapy and include which symptoms, which may indicate a need to check the INR? *(Select all that apply.)* **(416)**
    1. Black tarry stools
    2. Nosebleeds
    3. Claudication
    4. Petechiae
    5. Coffee-ground or blood-tinged vomitus

29. The nurse who is preparing to start a patient on IV heparin as prescribed knows that which procedures need to be done to ensure the correct dose is administered? *(Select all that apply.)* **(414)**
    1. Assess for signs of bleeding.
    2. Use a programmable infusion pump for the infusion.
    3. Anticipate the dose will be 70–100 units/kg/hour for the infusion.
    4. Ask another nurse to check calculations and the proper heparin strength.
    5. Monitor the patient for hematocrit, platelet counts, and aPTT levels.

30. A prescription for subcutaneous heparin was received by the nurse, who will prepare and administer the drug after reviewing which precautions? *(Select all that apply.)* **(414)**
    1. Plan to use the abdominal area.
    2. Avoid rotating sites of injection.
    3. Obtain the correct needle length—usually 1/2 inch.
    4. Avoid an area of 2 inches around the umbilicus.
    5. After injecting the drug, massage the area for 10 seconds.

31. When administering heparin, the nurse knows that this drug can be administered by which routes? **(413)**
    1. Orally, IM, IV
    2. Subcutaneously, IV
    3. IM, subcutaneously, IV
    4. Orally, subcutaneously, IV

32. It is appropriate to give only half the dose of protamine as an antidote for heparin, if it is given when? **(414)**
    1. At least 15 minutes after the heparin
    2. More than 30 minutes after the heparin
    3. In less than 30 minutes after the heparin
    4. After more than 60 minutes after the heparin

Describe the nursing assessments needed to monitor therapeutic response and adverse effects from anticoagulant therapy.

33. What therapeutic response does the nurse need to monitor when patients are on warfarin (Coumadin)? **(415)**
    1. Occult blood will be evident in stools.
    2. Urine may appear red, smoke-colored, or brownish.
    3. The prothrombin time (PT) or INR results will be within the recommended range.
    4. The skin and mucous membranes will have petechiae, ecchymosis, or hematomas.

34. Which adverse effect from warfarin (Coumadin) indicates that the patient is bleeding under the skin? **(415)**
    1. Anemia
    2. Petechiae
    3. Hematuria
    4. Thrombocytopenia

35. What measures are available for patients who have an excessively high INR from warfarin (Coumadin)? *(Select all that apply.)* **(416)**
    1. Administration of niacin (vitamin B_3)
    2. Administration of vitamin K
    3. Administration of naloxone (Narcan) as an antidote
    4. Administration of protamine sulfate as an antidote
    5. Administration of plasma or whole blood

36. What is the normal therapeutic range of INR for
    warfarin (Coumadin) therapy for a patient with a
    mechanical prosthetic heart valve? *(416)*
    1. 1.5–2.0
    2. 2.0–3.0
    3. 2.5–3.5
    4. 3.0–3.5

Drugs Used to Treat Heart Failure

Answer Key: Textbook page references are provided as a guide for answering these questions. A complete answer key is provided to your instructor.

MATCHING
Match the definition on the right with the key term on the left.

Term

1. _____ systolic dysfunction
2. _____ diastolic dysfunction
3. _____ inotropic agents
4. _____ digitalis toxicity
5. _____ negative chronotropy

Definition

a. having the ability to slow the heart rate
b. when the heart lacks sufficient force to pump all the blood
c. signs and symptoms include anorexia, nausea, and bradycardia
d. when the heart fails to relax enough between contractions to allow adequate filling
e. having the ability to stimulate the heart to increase the force of contractions

REVIEW QUESTIONS

Scenario: An 88-year-old male patient was admitted to the hospital with the diagnosis of exacerbation of heart failure. He has a history of coronary artery disease (CAD) with a stent placed in the past, pulmonary hypertension, hyperlipidemia, and asthma.

Explain heart failure in terms of the body's compensatory mechanisms.

6. The patient in the scenario has symptoms of systolic dysfunction of the heart causing decreased cardiac output and decreased tissue perfusion. What can the nurse expect to find upon assessment? *(Select all that apply.)* **(420)**
   1. Fatigue
   2. Peripheral edema
   3. Bradycardia
   4. Shortness of breath
   5. Exercise intolerance

7. What is the ultimate problem associated with diastolic dysfunction of the heart? **(420)**
   1. The peripheral vasculature develops stiffness.
   2. The symptoms of pulmonary embolism develop.
   3. The left ventricle becomes soft and boggy from being distended.
   4. The left ventricle becomes stiff and fails to relax, thus it does not fill adequately prior to the next contraction.

8. When patients are in heart failure, the kidneys respond to the decreased perfusion via the renin-angiotensin-aldosterone system, which stimulates the renal distal tubules to increase blood volume by what mechanism? **(421)**
   1. Excreting excess fluid
   2. Retaining sodium and water
   3. Increasing renin production
   4. Releasing epinephrine and norepinephrine

Identify the goals of treatment of heart failure.

9. The patient in the scenario has which underlying diseases that are treated to correct the heart failure? *(Select all that apply.)* **(422)**
   1. Asthma
   2. Hyperlipidemia
   3. Hypertension
   4. Thyroid disease
   5. CAD

10. The goals of treatment of heart failure include what outcomes? *(Select all that apply.)* **(421)**
    1. Prolongation of life
    2. Increasing intravascular volume
    3. Increasing exercise tolerance
    4. Being able to use only one drug to improve symptoms
    5. Reducing signs and symptoms of fluid overload

11. The patient in the scenario will be educated by the nurse on which lifestyle changes that are aimed at improving heart failure? *(Select all that apply.)* **(427)**
    1. Explore coping mechanisms the person uses in response to stress.
    2. Discuss adaptations needed at home to find positions for relief of dyspnea.
    3. Provide instructions for taking the blood pressure, pulse, and respirations.
    4. Discuss spacing activities of daily living to conserve energy and avoid fatigue.
    5. Provide food choices for a general diet with no fluid restrictions.

Identify the primary actions on heart failure of digoxin, angiotensin-converting enzyme inhibitors, angiotensin receptor blockers, the combination of a neprilysin inhibitor with angiotensin receptor blocker and beta blockers.

12. What are the desired therapeutic outcomes of digitalis glycosides (digoxin) for the treatment of heart failure? *(Select all that apply.)* **(431)**
    1. Improvement of dyspnea
    2. Improved tolerance of activity
    3. Tolerating oxygen therapy during rest
    4. Maintaining a serum digoxin level of 2.0 ng/mL
    5. Improved cardiac output resulting in improved tissue perfusion
13. The angiotensin-converting enzyme (ACE) inhibitors are used primarily in heart failure because they have what effect? **(428)**
    1. They increase the secretion of aldosterone.
    2. They increase sodium excretion in the kidneys.
    3. They reduce afterload by blocking vasoconstriction.
    4. They stimulate the heart to increase the force of contractions.
14. The drug class of beta-adrenergic blocking agents reduces blood pressure and is also used for heart failure patients because they are believed to have what effect? **(430)**
    1. They increase sodium excretion.
    2. They increase the secretion of aldosterone.
    3. They inhibit renin release to improve symptoms of heart failure.
    4. They stimulate the renin-angiotensin-aldosterone system.

15. The drug class angiotensin receptor blocker in combination with a neprilysin inhibitor will have what effect on patients with heart failure? **(429)**
    1. The combination drug will increase vascular resistance.
    2. The combination drug will work by different mechanisms to reduce preload and afterload.
    3. The combination drug will work by different mechanisms to slow the contractility of the heart .
    4. The combination drug will reduce circulating blood volume by inhibiting the secretion of aldosterone.
16. The phosphodiesterase inhibitor milrinone is available IV and used for short-term treatment of what for patients in heart failure? **(434)**
    1. Severe systolic dysfunction
    2. Severe diastolic dysfunction
    3. Borderline laboratory studies
    4. Therapeutic effects of ACE inhibitors

Describe digoxin toxicity and ways to prevent it.

17. The nurse will monitor which laboratory results of a patient who is on digoxin? *(Select all that apply.)* **(431)**
    1. Protime
    2. Digoxin level
    3. Serum sodium
    4. Serum potassium
    5. Serum creatinine
18. When a patient with heart failure on multiple medications is complaining of loss of appetite or any nausea or vomiting, as well as extreme fatigue, nightmares, and perhaps visual disturbances, the nurse should consider that what may be happening? **(432)**
    1. The patient is having dysrhythmias.
    2. The patient is experiencing digoxin toxicity.
    3. The patient is noncompliant with medications.
    4. The patient is experiencing worsening of heart failure.
19. In addition to hypokalemia, other clinical conditions that may also induce digitalis toxicity include: *(Select all that apply.)* **(432)**
    1. hypertension.
    2. renal disease.
    3. hypothyroidism.
    4. acute myocardial infarction.
    5. severe respiratory disease.
20. Before initiating digoxin therapy, the nurse will obtain baseline data such as what? *(Select all that apply.)* **(431)**
    1. Weight
    2. Vital signs
    3. Lung sounds
    4. Serum digoxin level
    5. Apical pulse for 1 full minute

21. The nurse will take an apical pulse for 1 full minute before administering digoxin and notify the prescriber if he or she detects what? *(431)*
    1. A pulse less than 60 or greater than 90 beats per minute
    2. A pulse less than 40 or greater than 120 beats per minute
    3. A pulse less than 60 or greater than 100 beats per minute
    4. A pulse less than 75 or greater than 120 beats per minute
22. The patient should be monitored for development of digitalis toxicity, which can be exacerbated by the presence of what electrolyte imbalances? *(432)*
    1. Hypokalemia and hypermagnesemia
    2. Hypokalemia and hypomagnesemia
    3. Hyperkalemia and hypomagnesemia
    4. Hyperkalemia and hypermagnesemia

Identify essential assessment data and nursing interventions needed for a patient with heart failure.

23. The nurse is teaching the patient in the scenario important health promotion measures and will emphasize which to the patient? *(Select all that apply.)* *(427)*
    1. Expect a short-term treatment.
    2. Continue with a lifelong treatment.
    3. Practice an exercise regimen.
    4. Follow a proper diet.
    5. Adhere to the drug therapy.

24. Which drug classes are used to treat patients in Stage A heart failure? *(Select all that apply.)* *(424)*
    1. Diuretics
    2. Statins
    3. Beta blockers
    4. ACE inhibitors
    5. Hypoglycemic agents
25. The six cardinal signs of heart disease associated with inadequate tissue perfusion include which symptoms? *(425)*
    1. Dyspnea, edema, chest pain, syncope, fatigue, palpitations
    2. Hypotension, dyspnea, chest pain, tachycardia, lightheadedness, hypokalemia
    3. Syncope, palpitations, tachycardia, atrial fibrillation, chest pain, edema
    4. Palpitations, atrial fibrillation, chest pain, syncope, edema, bradycardia

Drugs Used for Diuresis

Answer Key: Textbook page references are provided as a guide for answering these questions. A complete answer key is provided to your instructor.

MATCHING
Match the definition on the left with the key term on the right.

Definition

1. _____ a hormone that inhibits reabsorption of sodium in the distal tubule

2. _____ an excess of uric acid in the blood

3. _____ part of the kidney responsible for reabsorption of sodium and chloride

4. _____ dizziness, weakness, and faintness associated with a drop in blood pressure

5. _____ the part of the kidney tubule that forms a long loop in the medulla of the kidney

6. _____ a term used to describe excess fluid accumulation in the extracellular spaces

Term

a. edema
b. loop of Henle
c. aldosterone
d. hyperuricemia
e. tubule
f. orthostatic hypotension

REVIEW QUESTIONS

Scenario: A 74-year-old male patient was admitted to the hospital with a recent urinary tract infection. It was subsequently found that the patient had hyponatremia, with an acute kidney injury and history of hypertension and heart failure.

Identify the nursing assessments used to evaluate a patient's state of hydration and renal function.

7. When assessing a patient who is overhydrated, which assessment finding does the nurse expect to see? *(437)*
   1. Poor skin turgor
   2. Deteriorating vital signs
   3. Deeply furrowed tongue
   4. Neck vein distention

8. What are the classic signs of dehydration that the nurse will assess for and report? *(Select all that apply.)* *(437)*
   1. Weak pedal pulses
   2. Soft or sunken eyeballs
   3. Delayed capillary filling
   4. Shrunken or deeply furrowed tongue
   5. Skin turgor elastic with rapid return to flat position

9. A patient who has received IV fluids in excess of fluids excreted is likely to develop which signs? *(Select all that apply.)* *(437)*
   1. Peripheral edema
   2. Presence of crackles
   3. Sunken eyeballs
   4. Hypernatremia
   5. Mucous membranes glisten

10. When taking a history of a patient with fluid volume excess, the nurse should ask the patient questions relating to any history of heart disorders that contribute to fluid volume excess such as which conditions? *(Select all that apply.)* **(437)**
    1. Endocarditis
    2. Dysrhythmias
    3. Heart failure
    4. Myocardial infarction
    5. Patent foramen ovale (PFO)

11. The nurse listening to the lung sounds of a patient with fluid volume excess can expect which findings? **(437)**
    1. Clear breath sounds
    2. Crackles in the lungs
    3. Bronchial breath sounds over the trachea
    4. Vesicular breath sounds over the thorax

12. The nurse should be aware of which types of susceptible people who are at risk for the development of electrolyte disturbances? *(Select all that apply.)* **(438)**
    1. Patients who are pregnant
    2. Patients with massive trauma
    3. Patients who are receiving steroid therapy
    4. Patients with a history of cardiac disease
    5. Patients with a history of hormonal disorders

13. The nurse records accurate intake and output on patients who are taking diuretics and will record intake to include which fluids? **(438)**
    1. Liquid stools
    2. Ice chips in a liquid state
    3. The amount of vomitus
    4. Sputum that the patient coughs up

14. What laboratory studies should be performed whenever a diuretic is prescribed? *(Select all that apply.)* **(438)**
    1. BUN
    2. Sodium
    3. Potassium
    4. Creatinine
    5. Platelets

15. The nurse will assess which laboratory results for the patient in the scenario to determine the extent of kidney injury? **(438)**
    1. WBC
    2. Potassium and sodium
    3. BUN and creatinine
    4. Hemoglobin and hematocrit

Describe the actions of diuretics and their effects on blood pressure and electrolytes.

16. Which are therapeutic outcomes associated with diuretic therapy? *(Select all that apply.)* **(440)**
    1. Reduced edema
    2. Reduced blood pressure
    3. Decreased potassium level
    4. Improvement in the symptoms of fluid volume excess
    5. Decreased excretory load on the kidneys

17. The patient in the scenario is currently taking digoxin (Lanoxin), aminoglycosides, nonsteroidal antiinflammatory drugs (NSAIDs), and corticosteroids for multiple medical problems. Which principle does the nurse consider in monitoring this patient when bumetanide (Bumex) has now been prescribed? **(441)**
    1. The amount of digoxin will need to be increased.
    2. The potential for ototoxicity from the aminoglycosides is increased.
    3. The dose of bumetanide will need to be decreased when also taking NSAIDs.
    4. The use of corticosteroids and bumetanide may cause hyperkalemia.

18. A patient with type 2 diabetes mellitus and congestive heart failure is being treated with metformin (Glucophage), warfarin (Coumadin), and digitalis. The patient has a new prescription for bumetanide (Bumex). What adverse effects does the nurse watch for? *(Select all that apply.)* **(441)**
    1. Edema
    2. Dry mouth
    3. Fluid overload
    4. Orthostatic hypotension
    5. Electrolyte imbalance

19. The patient who has experienced vomiting and diarrhea is likely to develop which type of electrolyte imbalance? **(438)**
    1. Hyponatremia
    2. Hypernatremia
    3. Hyperkalemia
    4. Hypokalemia

20. When monitoring the laboratory values of potassium in patients taking diuretics, the nurse knows which is the normal value for potassium? **(438)**
    1. 135 mEq/L to 147 mEq/L
    2. 3.5 mEq/L to 5.5 mEq/L
    3. 1.6 mEq/L to 2.4 mEq/L
    4. 2.5 mg/dL to 4.5 mg/dL

21. Thiazides may cause or aggravate an imbalance in which electrolyte? *(Select all that apply.)* **(444)**
    1. Chloride (Cl−)
    2. Potassium (K+)
    3. Sodium (Na+)
    4. Magnesium (Mg+)
    5. Calcium (Ca+)

22. When thiazide diuretics such as chlorothiazide (Diuril) are administered, the drug is acting primarily on what part of the kidney? **(443)**
    1. The ascending limb of the loop of Henle
    2. The descending limb of the loop of Henle
    3. The distal tubules of the kidneys
    4. Enzymes in the kidneys that promote excretion of sodium and water

23. Carbonic anhydrase inhibitors are used as a mild diuretic, and also as an effective agent for which condition? *(440)*
    1. Glaucoma
    2. Hypothyroidism
    3. Gouty arthritis
    4. Peripheral neuropathy
24. Potent diuretics that act primarily by inhibiting sodium and chloride reabsorption from the ascending limb of the loop of Henle in the kidneys include which drugs? *(Select all that apply.)* *(440)*
    1. bumetanide
    2. metolazone
    3. furosemide
    4. torsemide
    5. acetazolamide

Explain the rationale for administering diuretics cautiously to older adults and individuals with impaired renal function, cirrhosis of the liver, or diabetes mellitus.

25. The patient in the scenario has the diagnosis of hyponatremia, and will most likely have to be supplemented with what? *(438)*
    1. Potassium
    2. Sodium
    3. Magnesium
    4. Chloride
26. When administering thiazide and loop diuretics to a diabetic patient, the nurse will need to monitor what lab results to prevent an adverse reaction? *(Select all that apply.)* *(444)*
    1. Sodium
    2. Potassium
    3. Blood sugar
    4. Hemoglobin
    5. Prothrombin time
27. A patient taking ethacrynic acid (Edecrin) is most at risk for developing dizziness, deafness, and tinnitus when he or she also has which condition? *(442)*
    1. Liver disease
    2. A hearing deficit
    3. Impaired renal function
    4. History of myocardial infarction
28. The patient with glaucoma who is receiving acetazolamide (Diamox) can expect which effect? *(439)*
    1. Insomnia
    2. Rapid heart rate
    3. Nasal congestion
    4. Increased urine output

29. The nurse discusses with the patient in the scenario which reasons for the medication furosemide (Lasix) to have been prescribed? *(Select all that apply.)* *(440)*
    1. "Lasix is the drug we give patients who have hypotension."
    2. "We are using the Lasix to treat your urinary tract infection."
    3. "This drug will induce hypernatremia to treat your hyponatremia."
    4. "The Lasix will help you get rid of excess fluid that your heart failure is causing."
    5. "Your hypertension and heart failure can be improved with the use of Lasix."
30. Thiazides used as diuretics have been shown to be effective in reducing edema and improving symptoms associated with which conditions? *(Select all that apply.)* *(443)*
    1. Renal disease
    2. Hyperglycemia
    3. Heart failure
    4. Hepatic disease
    5. Premenstrual syndrome
31. Which statements does the nurse include when teaching a patient about taking spironolactone (Aldactone)? *(Select all that apply.)* *(445-446)*
    1. "The purpose of Aldactone is to reduce your edema."
    2. "You should take your Aldactone before you go to sleep."
    3. "While you are taking Aldactone, avoid the use of salt substitutes in your diet."
    4. "You should be monitoring your blood pressure while on Aldactone, since it will lower your blood pressure."
    5. "One of the side effects from Aldactone is gynecomastia, which is irreversible."
32. The nurse gives which instructions to a patient who is on hydrochlorothiazide (HydroDIURIL) on how to reduce indigestion that the patient is experiencing? *(444)*
    1. "Always take this medication on an empty stomach."
    2. "It is best to take this medication with at least 8 oz of water."
    3. "This medication will cause gastric irritation no matter what you do."
    4. "Take this medication with food or milk to reduce gastric irritation."

Identify the nursing assessments needed to monitor the therapeutic response or the development of common or serious adverse effects of diuretic therapy.

33. If patients take salt substitutes while on spironolactone (Aldactone), the patient's laboratory results may indicate which electrolyte imbalance? *(446)*
    1. Hypokalemia
    2. Hyponatremia
    3. Hypercalcemia
    4. Hyperkalemia
34. What premedication assessments should be performed by the nurse on patients prescribed triamterene (Dyrenium)? *(Select all that apply.)* *(447)*
    1. Baseline weights
    2. Blood pressure
    3. Presence of edema
    4. Electrolytes and renal labs
    5. Need for hearing aids

35. The nurse observes the patient for signs of adverse effects from diuretic therapy mainly from electrolyte imbalance, which will be in the form of what symptoms? *(Select all that apply.)* *(447)*
    1. Tremors
    2. Nausea
    3. Nocturia
    4. Muscle cramps
    5. Altered mental status

Drugs Used to Treat Upper Respiratory Disease

chapter 29

Answer Key: Textbook page references are provided as a guide for answering these questions. A complete answer key is provided to your instructor.

MATCHING

Match the definition on the left with the key term on the right.

Definition

1. _____ a rebound of nasal secretions caused from overuse of topical decongestants

2. _____ drugs of choice for relieving congestion associated with rhinitis caused by the common cold

3. _____ a compound derived from an amino acid stored in small granules in most body tissues

4. _____ an inflammation of the nasal mucosa

5. _____ an inflammation of the nasal mucosa as a result of an allergic reaction

6. _____ a runny nose from nasal and lacrimal secretions

7. _____ a drug class that works by competing with the allergy-liberated histamine for H_1 receptor sites

Term

a. histamine
b. allergic rhinitis
c. antihistamines
d. rhinorrhea
e. rhinitis medicamentosa
f. decongestants
g. rhinitis

REVIEW QUESTIONS

Scenario: A 48-year-old male patient came into the clinic complaining of itchy, red eyes and frequent sneezing with nasal congestion. He was diagnosed with allergic rhinitis.

Describe the function of the respiratory system and list the common upper respiratory diseases.

8. The respiratory function of the nose is to do what to the inhaled air prior to its traveling into the lower respiratory airways? *(Select all that apply.)* *(449)*
   1. Warm
   2. Filter
   3. Humidify
   4. Detect odors
   5. React to allergens by sneezing

9. The upper respiratory tract is composed of which structures? *(Select all that apply.)* *(449)*
   1. Pharynx
   2. Tonsils
   3. Turbinates
   4. Eustachian tubes
   5. Lacrimal ducts

10. Which upper respiratory condition is actually a bacterial infection? *(451)*
    1. Sinusitis
    2. Common cold
    3. Allergic rhinitis
    4. Rhinitis medicamentosa

Discuss the causes of allergic rhinitis and nasal congestion and rhinitis medicamentosa.

11. What response does histamine release cause in the mucous membranes of the nose? *(451)*
    1. Stimulation of the olfactory cells
    2. Decreased ciliary movement
    3. Urticaria, redness, and edema
    4. Increased surface area of the nasal passages

12. The patient's symptoms in the scenario were probably caused by exposure to which allergens? *(Select all that apply.)* *(451)*
    1. Dust mites
    2. Viruses
    3. Pollens
    4. Grasses
    5. Animal dander

13. The nurse educating a patient on ways to treat rhinitis medicamentosa should provide the patient with which instructions? *(Select all that apply.)* *(452)*
    1. "The best treatment for this condition is to avoid it in the first place."
    2. "One option for you would be to work to clear one nostril at a time."
    3. "There are several treatment options available for you, but first it is important to understand the cause of the problem."
    4. "One option for you would be to completely stop taking the decongestant and work through the discomfort you will experience."
    5. "One option for you would be to switch to another decongestant—one that will not cause this condition."

14. A patient in the scenario was asking the nurse what would be recommended to treat his nasal congestion from allergy symptoms. What would be an appropriate response by the nurse? *(451)*
    1. "To eliminate your symptoms, you simply must avoid the allergen."
    2. "It does not matter what type of decongestant you use, they are all very similar."
    3. "You should avoid topical decongestants as their use could cause a rebound problem that is difficult to treat."
    4. "Only use prescription medications, as the over-the-counter medications often do not work for people."

Explain the major actions (effects) of sympathomimetic, antihistaminic, and corticosteroid decongestants and cromolyn.

15. What are the potential anticholinergic adverse effects of antihistamine therapy? *(Select all that apply.)* *(455)*
    1. Diarrhea
    2. Stuffy nose
    3. Dry mouth
    4. Blurred vision
    5. Urinary retention

16. Antihistamines such as fexofenadine (Allegra) are H_1 receptor antagonists and they work by what mechanism? *(455)*
    1. Blocking the H_1 receptor sites on the target cells
    2. Causing sedation and dryness of mucous membranes
    3. Constricting the blood vessels in the nasal passages
    4. Eliciting the production of a specific antibody against an allergen

17. What is recommended to patients with allergic seasonal rhinitis that does not respond to antihistamines? *(457)*
    1. It is recommended that they take NSAIDs.
    2. It is recommended that they take topical or systemic corticosteroids.
    3. It is recommended that they increase the dose of the antihistamines.
    4. It is recommended that they start taking cromolyn sodium.

18. Which statement does the nurse include when teaching a patient about the use of cromolyn sodium? *(458)*
    1. "Cromolyn sodium causes bronchodilation."
    2. "A 2- to 4-week course of therapy is usually required to determine clinical response."
    3. "Cromolyn sodium should be administered after the body receives a stimulus to release histamine."
    4. "Cromolyn sodium should be discontinued when the desired therapeutic response is achieved."

19. The nurse consults the prescriber before administering a sympathomimetic decongestant to patients with which conditions? *(Select all that apply.)* *(454)*
    1. Glaucoma
    2. Diabetes mellitus
    3. Hypothyroidism
    4. Allergy to shellfish
    5. Prostatic hyperplasia

20. When patients use nasal decongestants such as pseudoephedrine, they must be aware of the possible resulting hypertension, because of which action of sympathomimetic decongestants? *(454)*
    1. Vasodilation
    2. Vasoconstriction
    3. Bronchodilation
    4. Bronchoconstriction

21. The patient in the scenario also has hyperthyroidism, which prompted the nurse to caution the patient regarding the use of sympathomimetic decongestants because these agents will have what effect? *(454)*
    1. They stimulate the alpha receptors.
    2. They cause eye irritation and lacrimation.
    3. They have no effect on allergic rhinitis.
    4. They tend to produce stinging of the nasal membranes.

22. Which findings does the nurse typically assess in a patient experiencing a severe allergic reaction? *(Select all that apply.)* *(451)*
    1. Dry skin
    2. Urticaria
    3. Hypertension
    4. Bronchospasms
    5. Copious secretions

23. When a drug monograph says that a drug produces anticholinergic effects, the nurse anticipates that which symptoms may occur? *(Select all that apply.)* **(455)**
    1. Dry mouth
    2. Constipation
    3. Nasal congestion
    4. Urinary retention
    5. Blurred vision

Discuss the premedication assessments and nursing assessments needed during therapy to monitor the therapeutic response to and the common and serious adverse effects of decongestant drug therapy.

24. Decongestants are the drug of choice for which condition? **(454)**
    1. Allergic rhinitis
    2. Common cold
    3. Chronic sinusitis
    4. Anaphylactic reactions

25. What are important premedication assessments that the nurse will include for patients who starting on decongestants? *(Select all that apply.)* **(454)**
    1. Obtain baseline vital signs.
    2. Assess nasal and sinus congestion.
    3. Ask about any urinary problems, especially in male patients over 55 years.
    4. Review history for evidence of hypothyroidism or hypotension.
    5. Determine if the patient has glaucoma or cardiac dysrhythmias and consult the healthcare provider.

26. When teaching adult patients with blocked nasal passages about the correct order to administer their medications, the nurse will instruct them to do what? **(459)**
    1. Explain that they need to administer their intranasal corticosteroid before any decongestant.
    2. Explain that they need to administer a nasal decongestant just before the intranasal cromolyn sodium.
    3. Explain that they need to administer their antihistamine 30 minutes prior to the use of any decongestants.
    4. Explain that they need to avoid using a nasal decongestant; use their intranasal corticosteroid instead.

Drugs Used to Treat Lower Respiratory Disease

Answer Key: Textbook page references are provided as a guide for answering these questions. A complete answer key is provided to your instructor.

MATCHING

Match the definition on the right with the key term on the left.

Key Term

1. _____ ventilation
2. _____ diffusion
3. _____ asthma
4. _____ bronchospasm
5. _____ goblet cells
6. _____ bronchitis

Definition

a. the movement of air in and out of the lungs
b. smooth muscle constriction causing narrowing of the airways
c. specialized mucus glands of the respiratory tract
d. a common inflammatory disease of the bronchi and bronchioles
e. a condition causing inflammation and edema with excessive mucus secretion
f. the process by which oxygen passes across the alveolar membrane to the blood

REVIEW QUESTIONS

Scenario: A 75-year-old male patient was admitted to the hospital with respiratory failure secondary to pneumonia. After several days of being treated with steroids and antibiotics, he has stabilized on 2 liters of oxygen via nasal cannula. He has a history of chronic obstructive pulmonary disease (COPD), congestive heart failure, hypothyroidism, and rheumatoid arthritis, all of which are currently medically managed.

Compare the physiologic responses of the respiratory system to emphysema, chronic bronchitis, and asthma.

7. Which airway disease is characterized by restricted alveolar expansion due to loss of elasticity of tissue or physical deformity of the chest itself? *(463)*
   1. Reactive airway disease
   2. Obstructive airway disease
   3. Restrictive airway disease
   4. Resistive airway disease
8. How is asthma is best described? *(464)*
   1. A restrictive airway disease of the trachea
   2. A perfusion/ventilation disproportion condition
   3. A constrictive disease of the bronchi and bronchioles
   4. An inflammatory disease of the bronchi and bronchioles

9. Obstructive airway diseases, which are caused by narrowing of the airway, occur when which conditions are present? *(Select all that apply.)* *(462-463)*
   1. Edema
   2. Bronchospasm
   3. Decreased perfusion
   4. Excess mucus secretion
   5. Inflammation of the bronchial walls
10. What are examples of obstructive lung diseases in which the airway passages are narrowed and increased resistance to airflow occurs? *(Select all that apply.)* *(463)*
    1. Asthma
    2. Emphysema
    3. Acute bronchitis
    4. Pulmonary fibrosis
    5. Kyphoscoliosis
11. What is the process by which oxygen passes across the alveolar membrane to the blood in the capillaries? *(462)*
    1. Osmosis
    2. Perfusion
    3. Diffusion
    4. Ventilation

12. The respiratory tract normally produces thin, watery secretions to form a thin layer of fluid over the interior surfaces of the respiratory tract. Where does this fluid originate from? *(462)*
    1. The goblet cells and mast cells
    2. The cilia and alveolar membranes
    3. The mucus glands and serous glands
    4. The sebaceous glands and nasal mucosa
13. The important components of blood gases that nurses need to monitor that indicate overall pulmonary function are which values? *(Select all that apply.)* *(463)*
    1. Pa_{O_2}.
    2. pH.
    3. Pa_{CO_2}.
    4. HCO_3.
    5. Hgb.
14. Which component of blood gases measures the ratio of actual oxygen content of hemoglobin compared with the hemoglobin's ability to carry oxygen? *(463)*
    1. Sa_{O_2}
    2. Pa_{O_2}
    3. pH
    4. Pa_{CO_2}

Cite nursing assessments used to evaluate the respiratory status of a patient.

15. A nurse is assessing the patient in the scenario and listens to lung sounds. Which findings would the nurse report to the healthcare provider for further evaluation? *(464, 469)*
    1. Fine crackles throughout lung fields
    2. Diminished breath sounds at the bases
    3. Coughing up thin, white secretions
    4. Rapid, shallow breathing with O_2 saturation of 88%
16. During a respiratory assessment of the patient in the scenario, the nurse listens to breath sounds and monitors the respiratory rate, as well as what other symptoms? *(Select all that apply.)* *(469)*
    1. Appetite
    2. Mental status
    3. Pulse rate
    4. Signs of cyanosis
    5. Use of abdominal muscles during breathing
17. Which laboratory and diagnostic tests are also checked as part of the respiratory assessment? *(Select all that apply.)* *(470)*
    1. ABGs
    2. Chest x-rays
    3. Creatinine clearance
    4. Electrocardiograph
    5. Pulmonary function tests

18. The nurse needs to educate patients who have respiratory conditions on important health maintenance aspects, which include what instructions? *(Select all that apply.)* (470)
    1. Pulmonary hygiene
    2. Dietary and hydration needs
    3. Balancing activities with abilities
    4. Environmental control with filtration systems
    5. Use of abdominal muscles during breathing
19. The nurse was discussing the timing of the administration of medications for a patient with asthma. Which statement by the nurse is correct? *(471)*
    1. "It does not matter in which order you take your medications."
    2. "Take your steroid inhaler first, then your bronchodilator."
    3. "Take your bronchodilator first, then your steroid inhaler."
    4. "Take your bronchodilator first, then wait 2 hours before taking your steroid inhaler."
20. The nurse is explaining the different zones of a peak flowmeter to the patient with asthma and how to use it to assess when her symptoms are changing. The nurse recognizes that the patient needs further teaching after the patient makes which statement? *(470)*
    1. "The green zone is good, the yellow zone is warning, and the red zone is danger."
    2. "I can use the quick-relief medication when I notice that I am in the yellow zone."
    3. "The quick-relief medication and corticosteroids are used when I am in the green zone."
    4. "The peak flowmeter measures my peak expiratory flow and helps me determine how to manage my asthma."

Distinguish the mechanisms of action of expectorants, antitussives, and mucolytic agents.

21. Which drug is an effective cough suppressant and the standard against which other antitussive agents are compared? *(473)*
    1. Codeine
    2. Guaifenesin
    3. Ipratropium
    4. Acetylcysteine
22. Expectorants are those drugs whose action is to do what? *(472)*
    1. Relax the smooth muscles of the airway.
    2. Suppress the cough center in the brain.
    3. Increase the viscosity of mucus plugs.
    4. Enhance the flow of respiratory secretions, which promotes ciliary action.

23. The nurse was educating the patient on what to expect from mucolytics, and described them as having what action? *(474)*
    1. "These agents play an important role in the treatment of asthma to reduce inflammation."
    2. "These agents relax the smooth muscle of the tracheobronchial tree."
    3. "These agents may produce a goiter when used over an extended length of time in children."
    4. "These agents reduce the stickiness and viscosity of pulmonary secretions by acting directly on the mucus plugs to dissolve them."

24. The nurse gives a patient which instructions prior to the administration of an antitussive agent? *(Select all that apply.)* *(473-474)*
    1. "Be sure to drink plenty of liquids to keep hydrated."
    2. "Remember, this drug may cause you to become sleepy."
    3. "You need to describe the characteristics of your cough."
    4. "It would be wise to record your peak expiratory flow prior to use."
    5. "You need to make sure you have your nebulizing equipment for administration."

25. When administering guaifenesin (Robitussin) to a patient with bronchitis, the nurse expects that the drug will have what effect? *(472)*
    1. Dilate the bronchioles
    2. Thin the bronchial secretions
    3. Increase the viscosity of mucus secretions
    4. Increase the frequency of a nonproductive cough

26. The nurse will assess the action of acetylcysteine as working when the patient exhibits which symptom? *(474)*
    1. Kussmaul's respirations
    2. Increased nonproductive coughing
    3. Thicker and more viscous secretions
    4. Improved airway flow and more comfortable breathing

Describe the nursing assessments needed to monitor therapeutic response and the development of adverse effects from beta-adrenergic bronchodilator therapy.

27. What actions do beta-adrenergic agents have on patients with respiratory conditions such as asthma? *(475)*
    1. Bronchodilation
    2. Increase in respiratory rate
    3. Thinner respiratory secretions
    4. Decrease in peak expiratory flow

28. The patient in the scenario was given beta-adrenergic agents, and the nurse needs to monitor for which systemic adverse effects? *(Select all that apply.)* *(476)*
    1. GI disturbances
    2. Sedation, lethargy
    3. Bradycardia, arrhythmias
    4. Palpitations, tachycardia
    5. Restlessness, nervousness, anxiety

29. Which are short-acting beta-adrenergic agents that have a rapid onset and are used to treat acute bronchospasms? *(Select all that apply.)* *(477)*
    1. albuterol
    2. dipropionate
    3. salmeterol
    4. metaproterenol
    5. ipratropium

Discuss the nursing assessments needed to monitor therapeutic response and the development of adverse effects from anticholinergic bronchodilator therapy.

30. What actions do anticholinergic bronchodilator agents have on patients with respiratory conditions such as asthma? *(476)*
    1. They inhibit the inflammatory response in the bronchioles.
    2. They stabilize the mast cells to prevent the release of histamine.
    3. They block the cholinergic effect of bronchial constriction by the vagus nerve.
    4. They bind to the circulating antibodies in the blood, making them not as available to trigger symptoms.

31. What adverse effects from potent anticholinergic agents limit their use? *(Select all that apply.)* *(476)*
    1. Mydriasis
    2. Bradycardia
    3. Tachycardia
    4. Urinary retention
    5. Throat irritation

32. The following medications were prescribed for the patient in the scenario. Which ones are used to treat COPD? *(Select all that apply.)* *(478-479)*
    1. tiotropium (Spiriva)
    2. spironolactone (Aldactone)
    3. levothyroxine (Synthroid)
    4. indomethacin (Indocin)
    5. budesonide (Pulmicort)

List the lower respiratory conditions that use anticholinergic bronchodilators and corticosteroid inhalant therapy.

33. Which drugs enhance the effect of beta-adrenergic bronchodilators and inhibit inflammatory responses that may result in bronchoconstriction? *(478)*
    1. Xanthine derivatives
    2. Antileukotriene agents
    3. Corticosteroid inhalants
    4. Anticholinergic bronchodilators
34. Which are respiratory conditions that may be treated with any drug class—anticholinergic bronchodilators and corticosteroid inhalants? *(Select all that apply.) (478)*
    1. COPD
    2. Pneumonia
    3. Bronchitis
    4. Asthma
    5. Emphysema

35. Which patient condition is most likely to cause complications associated with beta-adrenergic bronchodilator therapy? *(475)*
    1. Asthma
    2. Pneumonia
    3. Diabetes mellitus
    4. Allergy to eggs
36. What instructions will the nurse give the patient who is started on systemic steroids for exacerbation of asthma? *(479)*
    1. "These steroids are given to allow easier breathing with less effort by decreasing pulmonary inflammation."
    2. "Your bronchodilator inhalant agents will be discontinued while you take these steroids orally."
    3. "Your corticosteroid inhalant therapy will be discontinued while you take these steroids orally."
    4. "The full therapeutic benefit from these systemic steroids may require up to 4 weeks of therapy for maximum benefit."

Drugs Used to Treat Oral Disorders

chapter
31

Answer Key: Textbook page references are provided as a guide for answering these questions. A complete answer key is provided to your instructor.

Matching
Match the definition on the right with the key term on the left.

Key Term

1. _____ canker sores
2. _____ candidiasis
3. _____ plaque
4. _____ gingivitis
5. _____ halitosis
6. _____ xerostomia
7. _____ mucositis

Definition

a. a painful inflammation of the mucous membranes of the mouth
b. an oral fungal infection
c. a condition in which the flow of saliva is decreased or completely stopped
d. oral lesions usually gray to whitish-yellow with a red halo of inflamed tissue
e. a whitish-yellow substance that builds up on teeth and gum lines
f. foul mouth odor
g. inflammation of the gums

REVIEW QUESTIONS

Scenario: A 52-year-old female patient arrives at the outpatient clinic with complaints of painful mouth lesions around her lower gums. The patient was diagnosed with canker sores and treatment was started to control the pain and facilitate healing.

Explain common oral disorders and their treatments.

8. The patient in the scenario asks the nurse in the clinic what could have been done to prevent these painful sores from developing. Which statement would be appropriate for the nurse to say? *(488)*
   1. "Everybody gets them, they will go away eventually; I would not worry about it."
   2. "Proper oral hygiene, such as brushing your teeth after eating, will prevent them."
   3. "You probably should have seen a dentist twice a year to prevent them."
   4. "The exact cause is unknown, but stress and trauma are precipitating factors."

9. The nurse was discussing with the patient who had xerostomia which treatment option? *(489)*
   1. "You can use mouthwashes to freshen the breath."
   2. "You can use a saliva substitute for this condition."
   3. "You can use topical analgesics to reduce the pain."
   4. "You can use an oral irrigation and proper oral hygiene."

10. Which situation can put patients at risk for the development of xerostomia? *(489)*
    1. Eating a meal with a lot of garlic
    2. Taking oral analgesics
    3. Rinsing with saline
    4. Smoking and mouth-breathing

11. Which mouth disorder is common in infants, pregnant women, and debilitated patients and is characterized by white milk-curd–appearing plaques attached to the oral mucosa? *(488)*
    1. Gingivitis
    2. Candidiasis
    3. Mucositis
    4. Xerostomia

Describe therapy used for oral health.

12. The patient in the scenario asks the nurse what she can do to minimize the pain from the canker sores. Which statement would be appropriate for the nurse to say? *(Select all that apply.)* ***(489)***
    1. "You can use any over-the-counter mouthwash to prevent halitosis."
    2. "You could place an aspirin on the lesion for pain relief."
    3. "Rinsing with saline may be soothing and can be done before you apply the medication."
    4. "You can expect that the canker sore will last for 3-5 days but you will have a scar."
    5. "If you apply the topical pain-relieving medication before eating or brushing your teeth, it may decrease the pain caused by these activities."

13. Patients who are being treated for cold sores should be taught by the nurse to do which treatment option? *(Select all that apply.)* ***(489)***
    1. Use saline rinses.
    2. Keep the mouth moist.
    3. Gently wash the cold sore with soap and water.
    4. Use highly astringent products on the sores.
    5. Allow the cold sore to dry so cracking can occur.

14. When discussing ways to prevent or treat halitosis, the nurse explains to a patient which measures to take? *(Select all that apply.)* ***(490)***
    1. Flossing regularly
    2. Using mouthwashes
    3. Brushing at least twice a day
    4. Applying Vaseline to the lips
    5. Taking antifungal medications

15. Proper oral hygiene of brushing twice a day should be taught to patients to prevent what disorder? ***(492)***
    1. Sinusitis
    2. Xerostomia
    3. Dental caries
    4. Canker sores

Identify nursing assessments and interventions associated with the treatment of mucositis.

16. Nurses need to perform an oral assessment in patients susceptible to mouth disorders to detect any abnormal findings such as what? *(Select all that apply.)* ***(490)***
    1. Well-fitting dentures
    2. Red, swollen gum line
    3. Pink, moist mucous membranes
    4. White patches over the tongue
    5. Teeth coated with food particles

17. Which action is most effective in providing a patient with relief of symptoms caused by mucositis? ***(491)***
    1. Avoiding exposure to the sun
    2. Applying amlexanox (Aphthasol) before meals
    3. Using commercially prepared mouthwash with alcohol
    4. Using 1 tablespoon of salt or hydrogen peroxide or 1/2 teaspoon of baking soda in 8 oz of water as a mouthwash

18. A patient has severe grade 3 mucositis as determined by the World Health Organization Oral Mucositis Scale. Which pain medications may be prescribed for the patient to treat oral mucositis? *(Select all that apply.)* ***(490)***
    1. Viscous lidocaine 2%
    2. Sucralfate suspension
    3. Milk of Magnesia rinses
    4. Nystatin liquid as a swish and swallow
    5. Aspirin tablet allowed to dissolve on the ulcers

19. How long does it take for mucositis to occur after a patient receives chemotherapy? ***(489)***
    1. 5-7 days
    2. 8-10 days
    3. 12-14 days
    4. 18-20 days

Drugs Used to Treat Gastroesophageal Reflux and Peptic Ulcer Diseases

chapter
32

Answer Key: Textbook page references are provided as a guide for answering these questions. A complete answer key is provided to your instructor.

MATCHING

Match the definition on the right with the key term on the left.

Key Term

1. _____ gastroesophageal reflux disease (GERD)
2. _____ peptic ulcer disease (PUD)
3. _____ *Helicobacter pylori*
4. _____ heartburn
5. _____ mucus cells
6. _____ parietal cells
7. _____ chief cells
8. _____ hydrochloric acid

Definition

a. secretory cells of the stomach that secrete hydrochloric acid
b. acid indigestion
c. secretory cells of the stomach that secrete pepsinogen
d. symptoms include epigastric pain noted when the stomach is empty
e. bacteria that are able to live below the mucus barrier of the stomach
f. the reflux of gastric secretions up into the esophagus
g. activates pepsinogen to pepsin providing the optimal pH
h. secretory cells of the stomach that secrete mucus

REVIEW QUESTIONS

Scenario: A 38-year-old male patient came into the clinic with complaints of acid indigestion and reflux and was diagnosed with GERD and prescribed an H$_2$ antagonist and an antacid.

Describe the physiology of the stomach.

9. What are the major functions of the stomach? *(Select all that apply.)* **(495)**
   1. Storing food
   2. Mixing food
   3. Maintaining a pH of 6
   4. Absorbing nutrients
   5. Emptying food into the small intestine
10. Which secretory cells line the stomach and secrete pepsinogen? **(495)**
    1. Parietal cells
    2. Chief cells
    3. Mucus cells
    4. Goblet cells

11. How are the parietal cells stimulated to produce hydrochloric acid in the stomach? **(495)**
    1. By the presence of gastrin
    2. By the presence of saliva
    3. By the presence of histamine
    4. By acetylcholine-stimulating cholinergic nerve fibers

Cite common stomach disorders that require drug therapy.

12. The patient in the scenario was given appropriate treatment for his GERD, but he could also have been prescribed which classes of agents? *(Select all that apply.)* **(497)**
    1. Coating agents
    2. Proton pump inhibitors
    3. Prokinetic agents
    4. Nonsteroidal antiinflammatory drugs
    5. Beta-adrenergic blocking agents
13. Which of these stomach disorders are treated with proton pump inhibitors? *(Select all that apply.)* **(503)**
    1. GERD
    2. Severe esophagitis
    3. Pyloric stenosis
    4. Hiatal hernia
    5. Gastric and duodenal ulcers

14. Patients with gastroparesis are sometimes given which drug to stimulate gastric emptying and intestinal transit? *(505)*
    1. cimetidine
    2. omeprazole
    3. sucralfate
    4. metoclopramide

Identify factors that prevent breakdown of the body's normal defense barriers resulting in ulcer formation.

15. One of the known causes of peptic ulcer disease is an infection in the mucosal wall of the stomach caused by which organism? *(496)*
    1. *Escherichia coli*
    2. *Helicobacter pylori*
    3. *Streptococcus viridans*
    4. *Staphylococcus aureus*

16. Patients older than 65 years with ulcer disease usually present with which symptoms? *(Select all that apply.)* *(499)*
    1. Weight loss
    2. Anorexia
    3. Dizziness
    4. Vague abdominal discomfort
    5. Burning in the epigastric region

17. What are the risk factors that increase the likelihood of peptic ulcer disease? *(Select all that apply.)* *(496)*
    1. Cigarette smoking
    2. Spicy foods and alcohol
    3. An infection in the stomach lining
    4. Excessive parietal cells secreting too much hydrochloric acid
    5. Injury to the mucosal lining of the stomach by NSAIDs

Discuss the drug classifications and actions used to treat stomach disorders.

18. Which class of medications is used in the treatment of peptic ulcer disease because it will inhibit gastric secretion of hydrochloric acid by inhibiting the hydrogen ion pump of the parietal cells? *(503)*
    1. Antacids
    2. Coating agents
    3. Proton pump inhibitors
    4. Histamine receptor antagonists

19. Which drug is a gastric stimulant that works by increasing stomach contractions, relaxing the pyloric valve, and increasing peristalsis, as well as working as an antiemetic? *(505)*
    1. lansoprazole (Prevacid)
    2. ranitidine (Zantac)
    3. metoclopramide (Reglan)
    4. misoprostol (Cytotec)

20. Which agents are used in the treatment of GERD and PUD for preventing and treating stress ulcers in critically ill patients by decreasing the volume of acid secretion causing the pH of the stomach to rise? *(500)*
    1. Antacids
    2. Coating agents
    3. Proton pump inhibitors
    4. Histamine receptor antagonists

Identify interventions that incorporate pharmacologic and nonpharmacologic treatments for an individual with stomach disorders.

21. Which statement does the nurse include when teaching a patient about antacid therapy for the treatment of peptic ulcer disease? *(499)*
    1. "Antacids take at least 6 weeks to become effective."
    2. "Excessive use of magnesium antacids results in constipation."
    3. "Antacid tablets do not contain enough antacid to be effective in treating this disease."
    4. "A common complaint of patients using large quantities of calcium carbonate antacids is diarrhea."

22. A patient with a history of chronic renal failure is on high-dose cimetidine (Tagamet) therapy for the treatment of a duodenal ulcer. It is most important for the nurse to assess the patient for which adverse effect of this therapy? *(501)*
    1. Diarrhea
    2. Dizziness
    3. Constipation
    4. Disorientation

23. When teaching the patient in the scenario about the use of antacids as part of the treatment for GERD, which statements does the nurse include? *(Select all that apply.)* *(499)*
    1. "Maalox is an example of a low-sodium antacid."
    2. "Use of an antacid with large amounts of magnesium usually results in constipation."
    3. "Calcium carbonate and sodium bicarbonate may cause rebound hyperacidity."
    4. "Patients with renal failure should not use large quantities of antacids containing magnesium."
    5. "Antacid tablets should be used only for patients with occasional indigestion or heartburn."

Drugs Used to Treat Nausea and Vomiting

Answer Key: Textbook page references are provided as a guide for answering these questions. A complete answer key is provided to your instructor.

MATCHING

Match the drug class on the left with the action of the drugs on the right.

Drug Class

1. _____ dopamine antagonists
2. _____ serotonin antagonists
3. _____ anticholinergic agents
4. _____ corticosteroids
5. _____ benzodiazepines
6. _____ cannabinoids
7. _____ neurokinin-1 receptor antagonists

Drug Action

a. act through several mechanisms to inhibit pathways to the VC with no dopamine antagonist effect
b. unknown mechanism of action, but other effects such as mood elevation and increased appetite may help
c. inhibit dopamine receptors that are part of the pathway to the VC
d. blocks the effects of substance P in the CNS and has no affinity for serotonin, dopamine, or corticosteroid receptors
e. counterbalance the excessive amounts of acetylcholine present at the CTZ and the VC
f. using a combination of effects such as sedation, reducing anxiety, and possibly depression of the VC
g. block the receptors of the 5-HT3 type located in the CTZ of the medulla

REVIEW QUESTIONS

Scenario: A 26-year-old pregnant woman came to the outpatient clinic complaining about severe persistent vomiting for the past several weeks. She states that it is impossible to keep anything down and now she is getting weak.

Describe the six common causes of nausea and vomiting.

8. Nausea and vomiting symptoms associated with motion sickness are thought to result from stimulation of what? *(509)*
   1. The diaphragm
   2. The cerebral cortex
   3. The labyrinth system of the ear
   4. The sensory receptors on the tongue and soft palate

9. The nurse knows that the six most common causes of nausea and vomiting include what? *(509-510)*
   1. Postoperative nausea and vomiting (PONV), chemotherapy-induced nausea and vomiting (CINV), radiation-induced nausea and vomiting (RINV), motion sickness, psychogenic, and pregnancy
   2. Pregnancy, PONV, CINV, COPD, RINV, motion sickness, and psychogenic
   3. RINV, motion sickness, PONV, pregnancy, CINV, and HTN
   4. PONV, CINV, motion sickness, pregnancy, psychogenic, and CVA

10. The patient in the scenario has which condition in which starvation, dehydration, and acidosis are superimposed on the vomiting, requiring hospitalization? *(510)*
    1. Drug toxicity
    2. Regurgitation
    3. Delayed emesis
    4. Hyperemesis gravidarum

11. Patients who have cancer and are undergoing treatment with gamma rays and chemotherapy may develop the adverse effect of nausea and vomiting, which is called what? *(Select all that apply.)* **(510)**
    1. Delayed emesis
    2. Psychogenic vomiting
    3. CINV
    4. PONV
    5. RINV

Discuss the three types of nausea associated with chemotherapy and the nursing considerations.

12. Chemotherapy and radiation therapy used for cancer treatment are associated with different types of adverse effects. Nausea and vomiting top the list as the most unpleasant, which can trigger a conditioned response by the sight of the clinic or hospital known as what? **(510)**
    1. Delayed emesis
    2. Regurgitation
    3. Hyperemesis gravidarum
    4. Anticipatory nausea and vomiting

13. What are the various ways that patients are treated with antiemetics to prevent CINV? *(Select all that apply.)* **(512)**
    1. Patients are given a combination of antiemetic agents.
    2. Patients are given the least emetogenic agent for chemotherapy.
    3. Patients are administered antiemetics prior to chemotherapy.
    4. Patients are encouraged to use over-the-counter herbal supplements for treatment.
    5. Patients are to continue antiemetic therapy for several weeks following chemotherapy.

14. Which antineoplastic agents are considered a high emetic risk (> 90%)? *(Select all that apply.)* **(510)**
    1. carmustine
    2. carboplatin
    3. cetuximab
    4. cisplatin
    5. cladribine

15. The nurse explained to the patient who recently underwent radiation therapy about which factors that influence RINV? *(Select all that apply.)* **(511)**
    1. The treatment site
    2. The field exposure
    3. The dose of radiation delivered
    4. The number of cancer cells radiated
    5. The previous development of nausea and vomiting

Identify the therapeutic classes of antiemetics.

16. The nurse was talking with a patient who mentioned he heard that marijuana is used for nausea now and would like some for his symptoms. What would be the best response by the nurse? **(523)**
    1. "You cannot have any marijuana. It is illegal."
    2. "I will have to ask your doctor if it would be okay for you to have any."
    3. "I heard it does not really help patients who are nauseated. I would not recommend it."
    4. "The active ingredient in marijuana has been made into a medication that your doctor may prescribe for you."

17. Most antiemetic agents used to reduce nausea and vomiting from motion sickness are chemically related to what? **(511)**
    1. Ginger
    2. Analgesics
    3. Antihistamines
    4. Ginkgo biloba

18. Which antiemetic medications would be of benefit to give to the patient in the scenario? *(Select all that apply.)* **(512)**
    1. Benzodiazepines (e.g., lorazepam, diazepam)
    2. Corticosteroids (e.g., dexamethasone)
    3. Antihistamines (e.g., diphenhydramine, meclizine)
    4. Phenothiazines (e.g., promethazine, prochlorperazine)
    5. Serotonin antagonists (e.g., ondansetron)

Discuss the scheduling of antiemetics for maximum benefit.

19. The nurse is educating a patient prescribed diphenhydramine (Benadryl) for motion sickness, and knows the patient needs more teaching after hearing which response? **(522)**
    1. "I understand that I should not drive a car after taking this."
    2. "This drug has fewer side effects than promethazine."
    3. "I will call my provider if I notice that I am starting to have trouble urinating."
    4. "For the best effect from this drug, I need to take it prior to travel by plane."

20. For patients undergoing chemotherapy, the nurse knows that if the acute emesis and nausea are controlled completely, the possibility of what is decreased significantly? **(512)**
    1. Motion sickness
    2. Delayed emesis
    3. Psychogenic vomiting
    4. Hyperemesis gravidarum

21. When should antiemetic agents be administered to be considered most effective? **(514)**
    1. It does not matter
    2. Before the onset of nausea
    3. After nausea has occurred
    4. After vomiting has occurred

Drugs Used to Treat Constipation and Diarrhea

Answer Key: Textbook page references are provided as a guide for answering these questions. A complete answer key is provided to your instructor.

MATCHING
Match the drug class on the left with the action of the drugs on the right.

Drug Class

1. _____ stimulant laxatives
2. _____ osmotic laxatives
3. _____ saline laxatives
4. _____ lubricant laxatives
5. _____ bulk-forming laxatives
6. _____ stool softeners
7. _____ peripheral opioid antagonists

Drug Action

a. bind to opioid receptors in the GI tract, inhibiting the constipating effects of opioids
b. lubricate the intestinal wall and soften the stool
c. cause water to be retained within the stool and increases bulk, which stimulates peristalsis
d. cause an irritation of the intestine that promotes peristalsis and evacuation
e. magnesium-containing products that stimulate muscle peristalsis to aid in evacuation
f. hypertonic compounds that draw water into the intestine from surrounding tissues
g. wetting agents that draw water into the stool, causing it to soften

REVIEW QUESTIONS

Scenario: A 72-year-old male patient admitted to the hospital with recent mental status changes, gastroesophageal reflux disease (GERD), and symptoms of gastric outlet obstruction was being managed with a nasogastric (NG) tube. He also had a history of Crohn's disease with a bowel resection resulting in an ileostomy and was experiencing high output from the ileostomy.

Explain the meaning of "normal" bowel habits and describe the underlying causes of constipation.

8. The nurse explaining to a patient what was meant by "normal" bowel habits uses which appropriate statement? *(526)*
   1. "Using laxatives or enemas daily should be just fine."
   2. "Daily bowel movements are necessary for good health."
   3. "Sometimes it is normal to have two or three bowel movements per week."
   4. "You need to start worrying about unhealthy bowel movements when the stool becomes soft and brown."

9. A patient asked the nurse for some advice on how to prevent constipation that was bothering him lately. Which response by the nurse would be appropriate? *(Select all that apply.)* *(527)*
   1. "Do you have any history of diseases of the stomach?"
   2. "What type of diet do you follow? One with plenty of fruits and vegetables and limited cheese and yogurt should help."
   3. "Tell me about your daily activity level. Being physically active helps eliminate problems."
   4. "Can you tell me about how much water you drink every day? It is important to keep well-hydrated."
   5. "Tell me about the medications you are taking. Certain types of drugs can cause constipation."

10. Which of these conditions may contribute to constipation for patients? *(Select all that apply.)* *(526)*
    1. Anemia
    2. Hyperthyroidism
    3. Hypothyroidism
    4. Tumors of the bowel
    5. Crohn's disease

Identify the mechanism of action for the different classes of laxatives, and describe medical conditions in which laxatives should not be used.

11. What is the mechanism of action of stimulant laxatives? *(529)*
    1. They draw water into the stool, causing it to soften.
    2. They add lubrication to the intestinal wall and soften the stool.
    3. They draw water into the intestine from surrounding tissues by means of hypertonic compounds.
    4. They act directly on the intestine, causing irritation that promotes peristalsis and evacuation.

12. Which statement does the nurse include when teaching a patient about the use of osmotic laxatives? *(529)*
    1. "These agents usually work within 8-12 hours."
    2. "Osmotic laxatives restore normal intestinal flora."
    3. "Osmotic laxatives work by making the stool softer."
    4. "Glycerin suppositories usually act within 15 to 30 minutes."

13. What is the mechanism of action of lubricant laxatives? *(530)*
    1. They increase peristalsis.
    2. They draw more water into the stool.
    3. They increase bulk in the stool to stimulate peristalsis.
    4. They lubricate the intestinal wall and soften the stool to allow a smooth passage of fecal contents.

14. Which statements about bulk-forming laxatives are true? *(Select all that apply.) (531)*
    1. They are used to relieve acute constipation.
    2. They are used to treat certain types of diarrhea.
    3. Adequate volumes of water must be taken with bulk-forming laxatives.
    4. They may be used in the treatment of patients with irritable bowel syndrome.
    5. They are generally considered to be the drug of choice for people who are incapacitated and need a laxative regularly.

15. What is the mechanism of action of stool softeners? *(530)*
    1. They lubricate the intestines.
    2. They stimulate peristalsis.
    3. They add bulk to the stool.
    4. They draw water into the stool, causing it to soften.

16. In which situations should over-the-counter laxatives not be used? *(Select all that apply.) (531)*
    1. Patients with constipation
    2. Patients with nausea, vomiting, or fever
    3. Patients with severe pain or discomfort
    4. Patients who have abused laxatives in the past
    5. Patients with success in the past using laxatives

Cite nine causes of diarrhea.

17. Which conditions predispose the patient to developing diarrhea? *(Select all that apply.) (527)*
    1. Anemia
    2. Hypothyroidism
    3. Crohn's disease
    4. Hyperthyroidism
    5. Enzyme deficiencies

18. Diet is an important consideration for patients who have developed diarrhea. The nurse educates the patient on which food items to avoid to prevent diarrhea? *(Select all that apply.) (527)*
    1. Spicy foods
    2. Fresh oysters
    3. Deep-fat fried foods
    4. Cheese and yogurt
    5. Drinking tap water when on vacation in another country

19. Which condition did the patient in the scenario have that is an example of a common cause of diarrhea? *(527)*
    1. GERD
    2. Crohn's disease
    3. Mental status changes
    4. Gastric outlet obstruction

Differentiate between locally acting and systemically acting antidiarrheal agents.

20. Systemically acting antidiarrheal agents such as loperamide (Imodium) work by which mechanism of action? *(532)*
    1. They promote the expulsion of formed stool.
    2. They absorb nutrients, water, and electrolytes and leave a formed stool.
    3. They increase peristalsis and GI motility via the autonomic nervous system.
    4. They decrease peristalsis and GI motility via the autonomic nervous system.

21. Locally acting antidiarrheal agents such as bismuth subsalicylate (Pepto-Bismol) work by which mechanism of action? *(Select all that apply.) (532)*
    1. They increase peristalsis and GI motility.
    2. They decrease peristalsis and GI motility.
    3. They absorb excess water to produce a formed stool.
    4. They reduce pain and irritation associated with diarrhea.
    5. They adsorb irritants or bacteria from the GI tract that cause diarrhea.

22. Which antidiarrheal agent has the potential to cause a hypertensive crisis when administered with a monoamine oxidase inhibitor? *(534)*
    1. loperamide (Imodium)
    2. bismuth subsalicylate (Pepto-Bismol)
    3. *Lactobacillus acidophilus* (Lactinex)
    4. diphenoxylate with atropine (Lomotil)

Describe nursing assessments needed to evaluate the patient's state of hydration when suffering from either constipation or dehydration, and identify electrolytes that should be monitored whenever prolonged or severe diarrhea is present.

23. The patient in the scenario was at risk for which condition? *(527)*
    1. Hyperkalemia
    2. Dehydration
    3. Hypernatremia
    4. Fluid volume excess

24. The nurse will need to monitor which laboratory values that may indicate a problem with malabsorption or dehydration for the patient in the scenario? *(Select all that apply.)* *(528)*
    1. Chloride
    2. Potassium
    3. Bicarbonate
    4. Blood sugar
    5. Alkaline phosphate

25. Assessments of the patient made by the nurse to determine if dehydration is present include checking which factors? *(Select all that apply.)* *(528)*
    1. Weight loss
    2. Excessive appetite
    3. Inelastic skin turgor
    4. Poor urine output
    5. Sticky mucous membranes

Cite conditions that generally respond favorably to antidiarrheal agents.

26. Which patient conditions generally respond positively to antidiarrheal agents? *(Select all that apply.)* *(532)*
    1. Severe constipation
    2. Following GI surgery
    3. Traveler's diarrhea
    4. Small bowel obstruction
    5. Inflammatory bowel disease

27. The patient in the scenario experiencing increased ileostomy output would likely receive which drug to inhibit peristalsis and reduce the volume from the ileostomy? *(533)*
    1. loperamide (Imodium)
    2. diphenoxylate with atropine (Lomotil)
    3. difenoxin with atropine (Motofen)
    4. Bismuth subsalicylate (Pepto-Bismol)

28. Which patient is most likely to benefit from the effects of a laxative? *(530)*
    1. 27-year-old who has colitis
    2. 65-year-old with gastritis
    3. 34-year-old paraplegic
    4. 49-year-old diagnosed with appendicitis

Drugs Used to Treat Diabetes Mellitus

chapter
35

Answer Key: Textbook page references are provided as a guide for answering these questions. A complete answer key is provided to your instructor.

MATCHING
Match the drug class on the left with the drug action on the right.

Drug Class

1. _____ alpha-glucosidase inhibitors
2. _____ dipeptidyl peptidase-4 inhibitors (DPP-4)
3. _____ thiazolidinediones
4. _____ biguanide
5. _____ meglitinides
6. _____ incretin mimetic agents (glucagon-like peptide agonists)
7. _____ sodium glucose cotransporter inhibitors
8. _____ insulin
9. _____ sulfonylureas

Drug Action

a. lower blood glucose by stimulating the release of insulin from the beta cells of the pancreas, but are nonsulfonylureas
b. a hormone produced by the beta cells of the pancreas, regulates metabolism
c. block the secretion of the protein located in the epithelial cells of the kidneys that reabsorb glucose back into the circulation
d. enzyme inhibitors that inhibit pancreatic enzymes used in the digestion of sugars
e. lower blood glucose by stimulating the release of insulin from the beta cells of the pancreas
f. decreases hepatic production by inhibiting glycogenolysis and gluconeogenesis
g. lower glucose levels by increasing the sensitivity of the muscle and fat tissue to insulin
h. prolong the life of active incretin hormones resulting in reduced hyperglycemia
i. enhance insulin secretion only in the presence of hyperglycemia, used for patients taking metformin

REVIEW QUESTIONS

Scenario: A 73-year-old female patient came to the outpatient clinic complaining that her left great toe was painful, swollen, and red. She has a history of type 2 diabetes mellitus, asthma, atrial fibrillation, peripheral arterial disease, gastric bypass surgery, and neuropathy.

Identify normal fasting blood glucose levels and differentiate between the symptoms of type 1 and type 2 diabetes mellitus.

10. Type 1 diabetes mellitus, caused by an autoimmune destruction of the beta cells in the pancreas, also has characteristics that differentiate it from type 2, such as what? *(Select all that apply.) (536)*
    1. Type 1 diabetes mellitus is thought to be auto-immune.
    2. Type 1 diabetes mellitus requires the adminis-tration of insulin.
    3. Type 1 diabetes mellitus can be controlled by eliminating sugar from the diet.
    4. Type 1 diabetes mellitus i is associated with increased frequency of infections and loss of weight and strength.
    5. Type 1 diabetes mellitus has symptoms that are characterized by polydipsia, polyphagia, and polyuria.
11. Diabetes mellitus is a group of diseases character-ized by what pathology? *(Select all that apply.) (535)*
    1. Impairment of insulin secretion
    2. Any plasma glucose level >126 mg/dL
    3. Defects in insulin action resulting in hypergly-cemia
    4. Fasting plasma glucose >100 mg/dL
    5. Abnormalities in fat, carbohydrate, and protein metabolism

12. Type 2 diabetes mellitus is characterized by which conditions? *(Select all that apply.)* **(536)**
    1. Type 2 causes an increase in glucose produced by the liver.
    2. Type 2 is caused by a decrease in beta cell activity.
    3. Type 2 patients often have an obese body type.
    4. Type 2 has a rapid onset over a few days to weeks.
    5. Type 2 is caused by insulin resistance, the reduced uptake of insulin by peripheral muscle cells.

13. Which statements does the nurse include when teaching health promotion activities to a patient with type 1 diabetes mellitus? *(Select all that apply.)* **(545-546)**
    1. "If you feel sick, cut your insulin dose by half."
    2. "Meal planning is important and getting consistent carbohydrates is recommended."
    3. "Self-monitoring of your blood glucose is advised when exercising."
    4. "Notify your primary healthcare provider immediately if you are unable to keep anything down."
    5. "Extra insulin is often needed to meet the demands of illness, so be aware of the development of hyperglycemia, which is common in patients with acute illness, injury, or surgery."

Identify the major nursing considerations associated with the management of the patient with diabetes (e.g., nutritional evaluation, dietary prescription, activity and exercise, and psychological considerations).

14. The medical nutrition therapy recommended for patients with diabetes includes which recommendations? *(Select all that apply.)* **(543)**
    1. Eliminating all sugar from the diet
    2. Weight loss is recommended for all adults with BMI > 25
    3. Use of the new system called the *consistent carbohydrate diabetes meal plan*
    4. Use of only the approved artificial sweeteners as sugar substitutes
    5. Limiting alcoholic drinks to two daily for men and one daily for women

15. The nurse was discussing how to count carbohydrates to determine the amount of insulin to be administered with each meal. Which statement made by the patient indicates a need for further teaching? **(543)**
    1. "I can have between 1500 and 2000 calories every day."
    2. "I should get approximately 45% to 65% of my calories from carbohydrates."
    3. "I should get approximately 20% to 35% of my calories from fat."
    4. "I should get approximately 25% to 45% of my calories from protein sources."

16. Patients with type 2 diabetes are managed by following which recommendations? *(Select all that apply.)* **(543)**
    1. Following a prescribed diet and exercise program
    2. Achieving weight loss to a near-ideal body level
    3. Taking insulin every day and testing blood glucose levels
    4. Reducing elevated cholesterol and triglyceride levels
    5. Taking oral antidiabetic agents when diet and exercise alone do not work to control blood glucose levels

17. The nurse is educating the patient in the scenario about activity and exercise, and because of her neuropathy, recommended which types of exercises? *(Select all that apply.)* **(545)**
    1. Walking
    2. Bicycling
    3. Swimming
    4. Rowing
    5. Treadmill

Compare the signs, symptoms, and management of hypoglycemia and hyperglycemia.

18. A nurse was discussing the symptoms and management of hypoglycemia with the patient in the scenario. Which statement by the patient would indicate further education is needed? **(546)**
    1. "When I start to feel hungry, get a headache, and my vision blurs, I know I am getting hypoglycemic."
    2. "When I start to feel hypoglycemic, I should drink some fruit juice with sugar added."
    3. "I can control the episodes of hypoglycemia by eating at regular times and watching what I eat."
    4. "I know I am getting hypoglycemic when I start to feel thirsty several hours after eating a large meal."

19. A nurse caring for a diabetic patient noted the following symptoms: increased thirst, headache, nausea and vomiting, rapid pulse, and shallow respirations. This could represent what condition? **(546)**
    1. Insulin overdose
    2. Hypoglycemia
    3. Hyperglycemia
    4. Paresthesias

20. Which drug classification when taken with insulin is most likely to induce hypoglycemia, and/or mask many of the symptoms of hypoglycemia? **(557)**
    1. Corticosteroids
    2. Benzodiazepines
    3. Calcium channel blockers
    4. Beta-adrenergic blocking agents

21. Which are considered causes of hyperglycemia? *(Select all that apply.)* *(546)*
    1. Overeating
    2. Vomiting
    3. Acute illness
    4. Infections
    5. Diarrhea

Describe the action and use of insulin to control diabetes mellitus.

22. Which type of insulin has an onset of 1-2 hours, peaks within 4-12 hours, and lasts from 16-28 hours? *(551)*
    1. Intermediate-acting
    2. Short-acting
    3. Rapid-acting
    4. Long-acting
23. When is the ideal time to administer rapid-acting insulin? *(549)*
    1. 30 minutes before a meal
    2. 30 minutes after a meal
    3. Within 10 to 15 minutes of a meal
    4. Immediately after a meal
24. What are the major advantages of insulin glargine and detemir? *(552)*
    1. They peak within 30 minutes.
    2. They are given in the morning for the best effect.
    3. They will decrease the blood sugar level rapidly.
    4. They do not result in large fluctuations in insulin levels.
25. The nurse is educating the patient in the scenario on the use of the rapid-acting insulin aspart while she is in the hospital and knows more education is needed after the patient makes which remark? *(549)*
    1. "This insulin has an onset of 1-2 hours and lasts 16 hours."
    2. "I need to have my blood sugar checked four times a day with this insulin."
    3. "The insulin aspart that I am receiving is a rapid-acting one that peaks in 1-2 hours."
    4. "So as I understand it, I will only be on insulin while I am in the hospital to control my blood sugar."

Discuss the action and use of oral hypoglycemic agents to control diabetes mellitus.

26. Which class of oral hypoglycemic agent lowers blood sugar in diabetic patients by increasing the sensitivity of muscle and fat tissue to insulin? *(558)*
    1. Meglitinides
    2. Thiazolidinediones
    3. Sulfonylureas
    4. Incretin mimetic agents

27. Which patient is most likely to benefit from treatment with sulfonylurea oral hypoglycemic agents? *(555)*
    1. Diabetic type 1
    2. Diabetic on 60 units of NPH insulin a day
    3. Diabetic type 2, not controlled by diet and exercise
    4. Newly diagnosed diabetic 18-month-old infant
28. Alpha-glucosidase inhibitors are an example of the type of oral hypoglycemic agent that works by lowering blood sugar in diabetic patients by what mechanism of action? *(560)*
    1. These agents increase the sensitivity of muscle and fat tissue to insulin.
    2. These agents inhibit digestive enzymes that result in delayed glucose absorption.
    3. These agents stimulate the release of insulin from the beta cells of the pancreas.
    4. These agents enhance insulin secretion and suppressing glucagon secretion from the liver.
29. The nurse realized the patient in the scenario was having difficulty with her diabetic management because her A1C level result was what? *(539)*
    1. 5.3%
    2. 6.0%
    3. 8.5%
    4. 4.0%
30. The patient in the scenario was being started on glipizide (Glucotrol). Which statement by the nurse would be included in the discussion of adverse effects from these drugs? *(555-556)*
    1. "If you develop a rash with itching, don't worry; it should get better eventually."
    2. "You will need to change your diet with these drugs and consume greater portions of protein."
    3. "You may experience nausea, vomiting, and abdominal cramps, in which case you must stop taking the drug immediately."
    4. "You may develop abdominal cramps and diarrhea, but these symptoms will resolve with continued use of your medication."
31. It is important for the nurse to inform female patients with diabetes that an alternative method of birth control should be used when taking which oral hypoglycemic agent? *(560)*
    1. miglitol (Glyset)
    2. glyburide (Glynase)
    3. ertugliflozin (Steglatro)
    4. pioglitazone (Actos)

Discuss the educational needs for patients with complications from diabetes (e.g., symptoms of microvascular and macrovascular complications).

32. What signs and symptoms of microvascular complications of peripheral vascular disease may diabetic patients develop? *(Select all that apply.)* **(547)**
    1. Pain with exercise and relieved with rest
    2. Urinary tract infections increase in frequency
    3. Reddish-blue discoloration may appear over legs and feet
    4. Temperature of the skin in the feet and legs may be cool to the touch
    5. Reduced blood supply to the extremities may result in intermittent claudication

33. The patient in the scenario had examples of complications from her diabetes. Which conditions are complications? *(Select all that apply.)* **(537)**
    1. Asthma
    2. Neuropathy
    3. Atrial fibrillation
    4. Peripheral arterial disease
    5. Cellulitis of the great toe

34. The major macrovascular complications of diabetes are associated with atherosclerotic disease of the middle to large arteries often leading to myocardial infarction and stroke, as well as what other complications? *(Select all that apply.)* **(537)**
    1. Retinopathy leading to blindness
    2. Ototoxicity leading to hearing loss
    3. Nonhealing ulcers leading to amputations of the lower extremities
    4. Renal disease leading to end-stage renal disease and dialysis
    5. Neuropathies leading to bladder incontinence and gastoparesis

35. The new diabetic patient needs instructions on how to manage diabetes, as well as any special equipment that is utilized, such as what? *(Select all that apply.)* **(548)**
    1. Syringes
    2. A computer
    3. A walker
    4. An insulin pump
    5. A self-monitoring glucose machine

Drugs Used to Treat Thyroid Disease

chapter 36

Answer Key: Textbook page references are provided as a guide for answering these questions. A complete answer key is provided to your instructor.

MATCHING

Match the definition on the right with the key term on the left. Definitions may be used more than once.

Key Term

1. _____ myxedema
2. _____ cretinism
3. _____ hyperthyroidism
4. _____ thyrotoxicosis
5. _____ hypothyroidism
6. _____ triiodothyronine
7. _____ thyroxine

Definition

a. congenital hypothyroidism
b. excess production of thyroid hormones
c. thyroid hormone
d. inadequate thyroid hormone production
e. hypothyroidism during adult life
f. excessive formation of thyroid hormones and their secretion into the circulatory system

REVIEW QUESTIONS

Scenario: A 48-year-old female patient came to an outpatient clinic complaining of increased fatigue and unexplained weight gain. She mentioned that she was beginning to have problems with constipation and felt cold all the time.

Describe the function of the thyroid gland.

8. Imbalance in thyroid hormone production may interfere with what body functions? *(Select all that apply.)* *(569)*
   1. Pulmonary function
   2. Cardiovascular function
   3. Thermal regulation
   4. Growth and reproduction
   5. Carbohydrate, protein, and lipid metabolism
9. The large, reddish, ductless gland located on either side of the trachea produces which hormones? *(Select all that apply.)* *(569)*
   1. Triiodothyronine
   2. Thyrotropin
   3. Thyroxine
   4. Thyroglobulin
   5. Thyroid-stimulating hormone

10. The hypothalamus and the anterior pituitary gland regulate the thyroid gland by secreting which hormones? *(Select all that apply.)* *(569)*
    1. Thyroxine
    2. Triiodothyronine
    3. Thyrotropin-releasing hormone
    4. Thyroid-stimulating hormone
    5. Thyroid-releasing hormone

Identify the two classes of drugs used to treat thyroid disease.

11. When drug therapy is prescribed for patients with hyperthyroidism, they may be given which drug? *(575)*
    1. liotrix
    2. levothyroxine
    3. liothyronine
    4. methimazole
12. The antithyroid drugs work by interfering with what? *(575)*
    1. The metabolic requirements of the body
    2. The release of thyroid hormones from the thyroid gland
    3. The formation of the hormones produced by the thyroid gland
    4. Release of thyroid-stimulating hormone from the pituitary gland.

13. The patient in the scenario needs to be started on a thyroid replacement hormone such as which drug? *(573)*
    1. methimazole
    2. propylthiouracil
    3. levothyroxine
    4. thyroglobulin

Describe the signs, symptoms, treatment, and nursing interventions associated with hypothyroidism and identify the drug of choice for hypothyroidism.

14. What focused assessments should be performed by the nurse for the patient in the scenario? *(Select all that apply.)* *(571)*
    1. Gastrointestinal—constipation
    2. Renal—decreased urine output
    3. Respiratory—rate and effort of breathing
    4. Auditory—presence of tinnitus
    5. Cardiovascular—pulse and blood pressure

15. A patient with hypothyroidism may require what dietary changes? *(572)*
    1. Increase in fats
    2. Decrease in calories
    3. Increase in calories
    4. Decrease in fats

16. The patient in the scenario was diagnosed with hypothyroidism and the nurse gave which instructions to her regarding this diagnosis and treatment? *(Select all that apply.)* *(572)*
    1. "You should take your Synthroid with food around lunchtime."
    2. "You will need to start taking thyroid hormones for the treatment of this condition."
    3. "You may find that you will be more comfortable in a warm environment."
    4. "You need to be aware of the signs of hyperthyroidism, which can be caused by too much thyroid medication."
    5. "The dosages of this thyroid medication start high and then gradually decrease in amount until you reach your daily maintenance dose."

Describe the signs, symptoms, treatments, and nursing interventions associated with hyperthyroidism.

17. Which disorders may cause hyperactivity of the thyroid gland that results in hyperthyroidism? *(Select all that apply.)* *(570)*
    1. Thyroid carcinoma
    2. Myxedema
    3. Graves' disease
    4. Nodular goiter
    5. Tumors of the pituitary gland

18. Which manifestation does the nurse expect to find upon assessing a patient who has been diagnosed with hyperthyroidism? *(Select all that apply.)* *(570)*
    1. Lethargy
    2. Constipation
    3. Weight loss
    4. Rapid, bounding pulse
    5. Nervousness and agitation

19. The primary therapeutic outcome for drug therapy for patients with hyperthyroidism is a gradual return to normal thyroid metabolic function expected from which drugs? *(Select all that apply.)* *(575)*
    1. liotrix
    2. levothyroxine
    3. liothyronine
    4. propylthiouracil
    5. methimazole

20. The nurse has been teaching a patient diagnosed with hyperthyroidism about proper nutritional habits to follow. Which patient statement indicates a need for further teaching? *(572)*
    1. "I will avoid chocolate."
    2. "I will drink decaffeinated cola."
    3. "If I get diarrhea, I will eat bran products, fruits and fresh vegetables."
    4. "I will eat a high-calorie diet, about 4000-5000 calories a day."

21. The patient in the scenario was on digoxin (Lanoxin) and needed to be started on levothyroxine (Synthroid) for the treatment of her hypothyroidism. The nurse explains which interaction between these drugs? *(574)*
    1. "You will most likely require a decreased dose of digoxin."
    2. "You will most likely require an increased dose of digoxin."
    3. "You will most likely require increasing dosages of Synthroid."
    4. "You will most likely have to adjust your dosages of Synthroid every week."

22. The nurse is instructing a patient recently diagnosed with hyperthyroidism on what activity is allowed. Which statement by the patient would indicate that further teaching is needed? *(572)*
    1. "I will need to pace myself with activities so that I do not get too tired."
    2. "I know that I should increase my activities every week even if I have pain."
    3. "If I feel weak and tired, I should not try to overdo it as far as exercising."
    4. "I understand that I should continue to be active but careful with overdoing exercise."

Discuss the drug interactions associated with thyroid hormones and antithyroid medicines.

23. Radioactive iodine-131 (^{131}I) is used in the treatment of hyperthyroidism because this drug will have what effect? *(575)*
    1. It will cause the thyroid gland to radiate a soft, warm glow.
    2. It will increase the circulating thyrotropin-releasing hormone.
    3. It will absorb all of the excess thyroid hormone that is circulating in the blood.
    4. It will be absorbed into the thyroid gland and destroy the hyperactive tissue.

24. When administering iodine-131 (^{131}I) to a patient, what actions does the nurse take? *(Select all that apply.)* *(575)*
    1. Avoids spilling the medication
    2. Changes the patient's bedding after each dose
    3. Wears latex gloves when administering the drug
    4. Adds the medication to water and has the patient swallow it
    5. Maintains hazardous medication precautions when working with the drug

25. Patients who require more than one dose of iodine-131 generally have to wait an interval of at least how long? *(575)*
    1. 1 month between doses
    2. 2 months between doses
    3. 3 months between doses
    4. 4 months between doses

26. A patient with dramatic weight loss and rapid, bounding pulse may be suffering from what disorder? *(570)*
    1. Cretinism
    2. Myxedema
    3. Hypothyroidism
    4. Hyperthyroidism

Corticosteroids

Answer Key: Textbook page references are provided as a guide for answering these questions. A complete answer key is provided to your instructor.

MATCHING

Match the brand name drug on the right with the generic drug name on the left.

Generic Drug Name

1. _____ fluocinonide

2. _____ budesonide

3. _____ mometasone

4. _____ hydrocortisone

5. _____ methylprednisolone

6. _____ prednisolone

7. _____ triamcinolone

Brand Name Drug

a. Kenalog
b. Vanos
c. Cortef
d. Prelone
e. Solu-Medrol
f. Nasonex
g. Pulmicort

REVIEW QUESTIONS

Scenario: A 75-year-old male patient was admitted to the hospital for respiratory failure and was diagnosed with pneumonia. He had a history of chronic obstructive pulmonary disease (COPD), osteoporosis, hypothyroidism, depression, congestive heart failure (CHF), coronary artery disease with previous bypass grafts, and rheumatoid arthritis. His medication list included levothyroxine, metoprolol, prednisone, duloxetine, acetaminophen, senna, and oxycodone.

Discuss the normal actions of mineralocorticoids and glucocorticoids in the body.

8. The adrenal gland secretes hormones that maintain fluid and electrolyte balance and regulate metabolism of carbohydrates, fats, and protein. These hormones are known collectively as what? *(578)*
    1. Aldosterone
    2. Glucocorticoids
    3. Corticosteroids
    4. Mineralocorticoids

9. The corticosteroids are used to regulate the body's metabolism. Which laboratory tests are to be monitored for patients receiving these medications? *(Select all that apply.)* *(579)*
    1. Hemoglobin
    2. Protime
    3. Glucose
    4. Potassium
    5. Sodium

10. The nurse has been teaching a patient with an exacerbation of rheumatoid arthritis about the use of glucocorticoids. Which statement by the patient indicates a need for further instruction? *(582)*
    1. "This drug has cured my disease."
    2. "This drug is relieving the inflammation associated with rheumatoid arthritis."
    3. "My fingers will not change back to normal shape due to this drug treatment."
    4. "I must be aware that I am more susceptible to infections when taking these drugs."

Cite the disease states caused by hyposecretion of the adrenal gland.

11. Which drug is given to patients who have a hyposecretion of the adrenal gland known as Addison's disease? *(582)*
    1. fludrocortisone
    2. dexamethasone
    3. methylprednisolone
    4. betamethasone

12. When patients are on the drug triamcinolone (a glucocorticoid), the medication may be in which form? *(Select all that apply.)* *(583)*
    1. Topical creams and ointments
    2. Tablets and injections
    3. Shampoos, gels, and oils
    4. Lotions and sprays
    5. Suppositories and foam

13. Glucocorticoids must be used with caution in patients with which disorders? *(Select all that apply.)* *(584)*
    1. Diabetes mellitus
    2. Peptic ulcer disease
    3. Upper respiratory infections
    4. Heart failure
    5. Mental disturbances

Identify the baseline assessments needed for a patient receiving corticosteroids.

14. What baseline assessments by the nurse should be completed for patients taking any type of corticosteroids? *(Select all that apply.)* *(578)*
    1. Daily weights
    2. Assess for dehydration
    3. Record temperature
    4. Pulse checks in supine and sitting position
    5. Orientation to date, time, and place

15. What is the priority assessment for the nurse to make when caring for a patient on fludrocortisone (Florinef) therapy for Addison's disease? *(582)*
    1. Allergic reactions
    2. Hyponatremia
    3. Hypokalemia
    4. Hypotension

16. The nurse is assessing the patient in the scenario taking glucocorticoids for the treatment of rheumatoid arthritis. Which findings are indications that the medication is exerting its desired effect? *(Select all that apply.)* *(582)*
    1. Pain relief
    2. Increased energy
    3. Relief of swelling
    4. Elevated sedimentation rates
    5. Normalization of preexisting joint deformities

17. Which signs of dehydration need to be assessed by the nurse when patients are receiving corticosteroids? *(Select all that apply.)* *(579)*
    1. Poor skin turgor
    2. Bounding pulses
    3. Peripheral edema
    4. Delayed capillary refill
    5. Sticky oral mucous membranes

Discuss the clinical uses and potential adverse effects associated with corticosteroids.

18. A nurse was teaching a patient with Addison's disease about the condition and how it is treated. Which statement by the patient indicates that further teaching is needed? *(580-581)*
    1. "I understand that I need to watch my weight and report significant changes."
    2. "I understand that my adrenal glands are not producing enough of the hormone needed to regulate water and electrolytes."
    3. "I know that when I go get my blood drawn, the most important test reported is the level of calcium."
    4. "I know I cannot stop taking these hormones unless I am under a healthcare provider's care."

19. Which types of illnesses or conditions are frequently treated with glucocorticoids? *(Select all that apply.)* *(582)*
    1. Allergies
    2. Bacterial infections
    3. Organ transplant
    4. Nausea and vomiting associated with chemotherapy
    5. Autoimmune disorders that require an immunosuppressant

20. What adverse effects does the nurse need to be aware of in patients who are receiving glucocorticoids? *(Select all that apply.)* *(584)*
    1. Hyperglycemia
    2. Hypoglycemia
    3. Peptic ulcer formation
    4. Increased susceptibility to infection
    5. Electrolyte imbalances and fluid accumulation

21. The nurse was teaching a patient about precautions necessary when receiving steroid therapy. Further education is needed when the patient makes which statement? *(583)*
    1. "I know I should not suddenly stop taking these medications."
    2. "I will need to get an identification bracelet to wear at all times."
    3. "I can expect that a weight gain of 2 pounds in 2 days is normal."
    4. "I understand that if I start to develop edema in my feet, ankles, or legs, I need to notify my healthcare provider."

22. The drug prednisone (a glucocorticoid) has an anti-inflammatory effect and is used for the patient in the scenario for which diagnosis? *(582)*
    1. Hypothyroidism
    2. Rheumatoid arthritis
    3. Depression
    4. Osteoporosis

Gonadal Hormones

chapter

38

Answer Key: Textbook page references are provided as a guide for answering these questions. A complete answer key is provided to your instructor.

MATCHING
Match the brand name drug on the right with the generic drug name on the left.

Generic Drug Name

1. _____ esterified estrogen
2. _____ fluoxymesterone
3. _____ conjugated estrogen
4. _____ norethindrone
5. _____ estradiol
6. _____ methyltestosterone

Brand Name Drug

a. Aygestin
b. Estrace
c. Premarin
d. Androxy
e. Methitest
f. Menest

REVIEW QUESTIONS

Scenario: A 29-year-old male with hypogonadism comes into the clinic complaining of muscle cramps, tremors, and feeling tired. It was determined that he was experiencing an electrolyte imbalance from his medication.

Describe gonads and their function.

7. The ovaries produce estrogens that are responsible for the maturation of the uterus, as well as which characteristics evident at puberty? *(Select all that apply.)* **(586)**
   1. Nail growth
   2. Hair growth
   3. Muscle mass
   4. Skin texture
   5. Distribution of body fat
8. Estrogens have which effects on the body? *(Select all that apply.)* **(586)**
   1. They cause fluid retention.
   2. They cause elevated blood sugars.
   3. They regulate protein metabolism.
   4. They impact the release of gonadotropins.
   5. They impact the release of gastrin in the stomach.

9. What are androgens used to treat? *(Select all that apply.)* **(591)**
   1. Hypogonadism
   2. Severe acne
   3. Palliation of breast cancer
   4. Androgen deficiency
   5. Wasting syndrome associated with AIDS

Discuss the body changes that can be anticipated with the administration of androgens, estrogens, or progesterone.

10. When androgens are given to females, what effects can be anticipated? *(Select all that apply.)* **(593)**
    1. Deepening voice
    2. Gastric irritation
    3. Clearing of acne
    4. Menstrual irregularity
    5. Growth of facial hair
11. The nurse is teaching a patient about the adverse effects of estrogen therapy. Which statement by the patient indicates a need for further teaching? **(588)**
    1. "Weight gain is a common adverse effect of estrogen therapy."
    2. "Breast tenderness is to be expected when I start this drug."
    3. "Low blood pressure is a common side effect of estrogen therapy."
    4. "If I experience any breakthrough bleeding between my menstrual periods, I will notify my primary care provider immediately."

12. The nurse is teaching the patient in the scenario about ways to minimize the adverse effects of androgen therapy, which include what suggestions? *(Select all that apply.)* **(593)**
    1. "You should drink 8-12 glasses of water a day."
    2. "You should chew and swallow the buccal tablet."
    3. "You should include weight-bearing exercises in your ADLs."
    4. "You should report any weight gain of more than 2 pounds per week."
    5. "You should notify the prescriber if nausea, anorexia, and jaundice occur."

13. The patient in the scenario is ordered testosterone gel every 24 hours. The nurse teaches the patient to rotate the application sites for the patch to which areas of the body? *(Select all that apply.)* **(592)**
    1. Hips
    2. Abdomen
    3. Shoulders
    4. Upper arms
    5. Scrotum

Identify the uses of estrogens and progestins.

14. Progestin therapy is used to treat which conditions? *(Select all that apply.)* **(590)**
    1. Severe acne
    2. Endometriosis
    3. Secondary amenorrhea
    4. Breakthrough uterine bleeding
    5. Hot flash symptoms of menopause

15. The therapeutic uses for estrogen therapy are to do what? *(Select all that apply.)* **(588)**
    1. Treat acne in males
    2. Treat osteoporosis
    3. Provide contraception
    4. Treat advanced prostate cancer
    5. Relieve hot flash symptoms of menopause

16. When is the use of estrogens contraindicated? **(588)**
    1. Postpartum
    2. During menopause
    3. During early pregnancy
    4. With advanced prostatic cancer

Compare the adverse effects seen with the use of estrogen hormones with those seen with androgens.

17. While assessing a female patient on estrogen therapy for birth control, which adverse effect does the nurse report to the healthcare provider? **(588)**
    1. Nausea
    2. Weight gain
    3. Breast tenderness
    4. Breakthrough bleeding

18. Which gonadal hormone therapy is used for palliative treatment of prostate cancer? **(588)**
    1. Thyroid therapy
    2. Progestin therapy
    3. Androgen therapy
    4. Estrogen therapy

19. The nurse is teaching the patient in the scenario to report which effects of methyltestosterone to the healthcare provider? *(Select all that apply.)* **(592-593)**
    1. Masculinization
    2. Gastric irritation
    3. Jaundice, anorexia
    4. Weight gain of more than 2 pounds in a week
    5. Nausea, vomiting, constipation, and lethargy

20. When patients are started on estrogen therapy, which drug interactions may occur? *(Select all that apply.)* **(588)**
    1. Rifampin and estrogens may cause jaundice.
    2. Insulin and estrogens may cause hypoglycemia.
    3. Warfarin and estrogens may result in risk for clotting.
    4. Thyroid hormones and estrogens may cause hypothyroidism.
    5. Phenytoin and estrogens may cause toxicity of phenytoin.

21. Which serious adverse effects may be experienced with progestins? *(Select all that apply.)* **(591)**
    1. Severe acne
    2. Depression
    3. Cholestatic jaundice
    4. Continuous headache
    5. Weight gain and edema

Drugs Used in Obstetrics

chapter
39

Answer Key: Textbook page references are provided as a guide for answering these questions. A complete answer key is provided to your instructor.

MATCHING
Match the drug name on the right with the correct usage for the drug on the left.

Usage for Drug

1. _____ used to inhibit premature labor
2. _____ used to include labor at term
3. _____ used to expel uterine contents
4. _____ used to induce ovulation
5. _____ used as a cervical ripening agent
6. _____ used in small doses in postpartum patients to control bleeding

Drug

a. misoprostol
b. dinoprostone
c. methylergonovine maleate
d. oxytocin
e. magnesium sulfate
f. clomiphene citrate

REVIEW QUESTIONS

Scenario: A 32-year-old gravida 1, para 0 was admitted after 38 weeks gestation to the local delivery unit in possible labor. After the initial assessment, the patient was noted to have high blood pressure, pedal edema, and hyperreflexia. The patient was diagnosed with preeclampsia and was started on a magnesium sulfate infusion.

Identify appropriate nursing assessments during normal labor and delivery.

7. The nurse needs to be aware of which potential obstetric complications in pregnant women? *(Select all that apply.) (596)*
   1. Infection
   2. Preterm labor
   3. Hypoglycemia
   4. Gestational diabetes
   5. Premature rupture of membranes

8. The nurse was discussing postpartum care with a new mother and knew that more teaching was needed after the mother made which statement? *(602)*
   1. "I understand that my baby will gain about 1 ounce per day until day 5."
   2. "I can take a mild analgesic 40 minutes before breastfeeding."
   3. "I know I need to continue to eat a well-balanced diet when breastfeeding."
   4. "If I note any foul odor from my vaginal discharge, I know to call my healthcare provider."

9. What are routine nursing assessments performed on pregnant women no matter what trimester they are in? *(Select all that apply.) (596)*
   1. Weight
   2. Blood pressure
   3. Vaginal exams
   4. Hemoglobin and hematocrit
   5. Fundal height and fetal heart sounds

10. Assessments of pregnant women include obtaining an obstetric history, which means the nurse asks about what? *(Select all that apply.) (596)*
    1. Previous live births
    2. Any cesarean deliveries
    3. Current medications
    4. Premature deliveries
    5. Spontaneous or therapeutic abortions

Discuss potential complications of preterm labor and when uterine relaxants and magnesium sulfate are used.

11. Which are primary clinical indications for the use of uterine stimulants? *(Select all that apply.)* *(605)*
    1. Suppression of lactation
    2. Induction of therapeutic abortion
    3. Induction or augmentation of labor
    4. Control of postsurgical hemorrhage
    5. Control of postpartum atony and hemorrhage

12. What are some reasons for the use of uterine relaxants on the pregnant uterus? *(610)*
    1. They are used to induce or augment labor.
    2. They are used to control postpartum hemorrhage.
    3. They are used to suppress the flow of colostrum.
    4. They are used to delay or prevent labor and delivery in selected patients.

13. Which assessment findings that the nurse obtained from the patient in the scenario would indicate that the magnesium sulfate infusion should be discontinued? *(611)*
    1. Absence of deep tendon reflexes
    2. Respiratory rate of 16 breaths/min
    3. Urinary output of 45 mL during the past hour
    4. Decrease in blood pressure from 180/100 to 150/90 mm Hg

14. What nursing action needs to be taken when a pregnant woman is in preterm labor? *(610)*
    1. Restrict fluids.
    2. Position the patient on her back.
    3. Administer uterine stimulants.
    4. Administer uterine relaxants.

15. What are signs of fetal distress? *(609)*
    1. Fetal heart rate 120–160 beats/min following any contraction
    2. Fetal heart rate >160 beats/min lasting less than 10 seconds after contractions
    3. Fetal heart rate 140 beats/min lasting longer than 15 seconds after contractions
    4. Fetal heart rate >160 followed by heart rate <120 occurring frequently following contractions

Describe when uterine stimulants are administered for induction of labor, augmentation of labor, and postpartum atony and hemorrhage.

16. The nurse assesses a patient receiving an infusion of oxytocin (Pitocin) to induce labor and determines the infant is in distress. Which actions does the nurse take? *(Select all that apply.)* *(609)*
    1. Turns the patient to the right lateral position
    2. Notifies the healthcare provider immediately
    3. Administers a bolus of magnesium sulfate
    4. Administers oxygen by nasal cannula or facemask
    5. Reduces the oxytocin infusion to the slowest possible rate according to hospital policy

17. The nurse was performing a postpartum assessment on a mother who was receiving oxytocin (Pitocin) therapy for control of bleeding and found the uterus to be boggy. What is the nurse's next action? *(610)*
    1. Massage the uterus.
    2. Administer magnesium sulfate.
    3. Slow the rate of the infusion.
    4. Call the healthcare provider immediately.

18. When working with patients receiving oxytocin (Pitocin), the nurse must assess for the development of water intoxication because oxytocin therapy causes which effect? *(609)*
    1. Hypertension
    2. Hypocalcemia
    3. Extreme thirst in patients
    4. Stimulation of antidiuretic hormone

19. List in correct order the steps to take for managing patients in preterm labor. *(598)*
    1. _____ Determine contraindications to tocolysis (i.e., placenta previa, fetal distress).
    2. _____ Monitor contractions and determine estimated gestational age.
    3. _____ Administer nifedipine and betamethasone.
    4. _____ Take vital signs of the mother and apply fetal monitoring.
    5. _____ Observe for cervical changes.

20. A patient is receiving magnesium sulfate to inhibit preterm labor. Which drug does the nurse have readily available if magnesium intoxication should occur? *(611)*
    1. Atropine
    2. Epinephrine
    3. Calcium gluconate
    4. Potassium chloride

State the actions of clomiphene citrate and the primary use.

21. Which drug is used to induce ovulation in women who are not ovulating because of low estrogen levels? *(612)*
    1. Misoprostol
    2. Magnesium sulfate
    3. Ergonovine maleate
    4. Clomiphene citrate

22. The nurse educating a woman who is taking clomiphene to get pregnant about precautions to take includes which statements? *(Select all that apply.)* *(612)*
    1. "This medication may result in multiple fetuses."
    2. "Clomiphene usually takes three or four courses before it is effective."
    3. "You need to take and record your temperature for 1 month after taking this."
    4. "Timing of intercourse is important for success, so make sure that this occurs during the time of ovulation."
    5. "You need to take the medication every day for 5 days and then wait to determine if ovulation occurs."

23. A patient who is taking clomiphene to get pregnant asks the nurse about timing of intercourse. Which is an appropriate statement by the nurse? *(612)*
    1. "Timing does not matter; this medication will work no matter what you do."
    2. "It would be best to have intercourse at the same time every day for a month."
    3. "Intercourse should be timed during ovulation, usually 6-10 days after the last dose."
    4. "You should time intercourse to occur when your temperature follows a biphasic pattern."

Identify the action and proper timing of the administration of Rho(D) immune globulin.

24. When is the recommended time of administration for Rho(D) immune globulin once the mother has delivered her baby? *(613)*
    1. Immediately after delivery
    2. Within 72 hours of delivery
    3. Only after the patient starts to hemorrhage
    4. Prior to discharge from the hospital

25. What does Rho(D) immune globulin do when administered to patients? *(613)*
    1. It prevents ovulation.
    2. It induces termination of pregnancy.
    3. It prevents postpartum gonorrhea infection.
    4. It prevents Rh hemolytic disease in subsequent deliveries.

26. The nursing assessments needed prior to administration of Rho(D) immune globulin include checking what? *(Select all that apply.)* *(613)*
    1. The Rh status of the mother
    2. The platelet count of the mother
    3. The Rh status of the infant
    4. The platelet count of the infant
    5. To determine if the mother is already sensitized

Cite education needed for care of the neonate, including erythromycin ophthalmic ointment and phytonadione administration.

27. The health status of the neonate is estimated at 1 minute and 5 minutes after delivery using the Apgar rating system, which assesses which parameters of the newborn? *(Select all that apply.)* *(599)*
    1. Heart rate
    2. Blood pressure
    3. Muscle tone
    4. Reflex irritability
    5. Color of body and extremities

28. Which procedures need to be attended to following the delivery of the newborn? *(Select all that apply.)* *(602)*
    1. Breastfeeding
    2. Eye prophylaxis
    3. Clamping the umbilical cord
    4. Determining an Apgar score
    5. Airway—suction with bulb syringe if needed

29. After birth, all infants have prophylactic erythromycin ointment applied to their eyes to prevent what? *(614)*
    1. Wilms' tumor
    2. Nearsightedness
    3. Pheochromocytoma
    4. Ophthalmia neonatorum

30. A new mother asks the nurse why her newborn needs a shot of vitamin K. Which is an appropriate statement by the nurse? *(614)*
    1. "All babies get this to prevent ophthalmia neonatorum."
    2. "The delivery may have caused an infection in your baby and this will take care of it."
    3. "This will help increase the amount of natural bacteria in your baby's GI system."
    4. "Newborns are often deficient in vitamin K and we want to prevent any bleeding issues."

Drugs Used in Men's and Women's Health

Answer Key: Textbook page references are provided as a guide for answering these questions. A complete answer key is provided to your instructor.

MATCHING

Match the term on the right with the definition on the left.

Definition

1. _____ pathogens commonly transmitted by sexual contact

2. _____ an enlargement of the prostate gland

3. _____ the consistent inability to achieve or maintain an erection sufficient for satisfactory sexual activity

4. _____ an abnormal, whitish vaginal discharge that can occur at any age

5. _____ a common bone disease of low mineral density which results in bone fragility and risk of fractures

6. _____ irregular periods, infrequent periods, and spotting between periods

Term

a. leukorrhea
b. sexually transmitted infections
c. dysmenorrhea
d. osteoporosis
e. benign prostatic hyperplasia
f. erectile dysfunction

REVIEW QUESTIONS

Scenario: A couple came into the clinic with a request to be tested for gonorrhea and described abnormal vaginal discharge and urethral discharge from the penis.

Identify important personal hygiene measures to educate women and men regarding prevention of the spread of sexually transmitted infections.

7. Which patient education instructions are important to review when discussing hygiene measures with the couple in the scenario to prevent the spread of sexually transmitted infection? *(Select all that apply.)* *(620)*
   1. Use latex condoms.
   2. Urinate after intercourse.
   3. Douching after intercourse is effective in preventing pregnancy and HIV.
   4. Practice abstinence during the communicable phase of any disease.
   5. Spermicides, sponges, and diaphragms are effective in preventing transmission of HIV.

8. Which of these sexually transmitted infections are reportable by the health department in every state? *(Select all that apply.)* *(620)*
   1. AIDS
   2. Syphilis
   3. Gonorrhea
   4. Chlamydia
   5. Herpes simplex virus

9. The nurse is educating the couple in the scenario regarding preventing the spread of sexually transmitted infections and determines that further teaching is needed after hearing which comment? *(620)*
   1. The man: "Next time, I can just use a condom."
   2. The woman: "We will need to be abstinent from sex until this infection clears up."
   3. The woman: "I know I need to get a routine physical exam including a pelvic and breast exam and a Pap smear."
   4. The man: "I know I need to get a routine physical exam including a testicular exam, but not a rectal exam until I am over 40."

Describe the major adverse effects and contraindications to the use of oral contraceptive agents.

10. Which adverse effect from the combination pill is of concern and needs to be reported as soon as possible? *(624)*
    1. Nausea
    2. Chloasma
    3. Weight gain
    4. Leg pain, chest pain, or shortness of breath

11. The minipill, which only contains progestin, is preferred by some women because of their history of which conditions that are aggravated by estrogens? *(Select all that apply.) (623)*
    1. Diabetes
    2. Depression
    3. Migraines
    4. Hypertension
    5. Hypothyroidism

12. Why is smoking while on the pill considered to be so risky for women? *(623)*
    1. The chance of pregnancy is increased.
    2. The possibility of breakthrough bleeding is increased.
    3. The pill loses its effectiveness after just one cigarette.
    4. The likelihood of developing a serious blood clot is increased.

13. Which type of combination pill is used for patients who have heavy menses with associated anemia? *(623)*
    1. Biphasic
    2. Triphasic
    3. Quadriphasic
    4. Continuous cycle

14. What precaution must be taken prior to starting oral contraceptives? *(623)*
    1. Obtain a list of past sexual partners.
    2. Ensure that the patient is not pregnant.
    3. Determine the sperm count of the male partner.
    4. Determine if any sexually transmitted infections have been contracted.

15. How does the minipill produce contraception differently from the combination pill? *(621)*
    1. By causing the cervical mucus to become thicker
    2. By inhibiting the release of luteinizing hormone
    3. By causing sperm migration to be inhibited by viscous mucus
    4. By blocking the pituitary release of follicle-stimulating hormone

Identify the patient teaching necessary with the administration of the transdermal contraceptive and the intravaginal hormonal contraceptive.

16. In teaching a patient about the use of norelgestromin-ethinyl estradiol transdermal system (Xulane), which statements does the nurse include? *(Select all that apply.) (626)*
    1. "Do not place the patch on your breast."
    2. "Trim the patch to best fit the area where you wish to apply it."
    3. "Apply the patch to the buttock, abdomen, upper outer arm, or upper torso."
    4. "Avoid lotions or creams on the areas of the skin where the patch is applied because the patch may not adhere properly."
    5. "If the patch is partially detached for less than 24 hours, try to reapply it in the same place or replace it with a new patch immediately."

17. A patient asks the nurse about what to do when she misses her period while on the NuvaRing. What is an appropriate response by the nurse? *(628)*
    1. "When you are using the ring, you will need to keep track of your periods and call if you miss one."
    2. "It is uncommon to miss a period while using the ring, but you will need to be seen by a healthcare provider if this happens."
    3. "Since missing one period is not uncommon, continue on the same cycle, but if two consecutive periods are missed a pregnancy test is needed."
    4. "Missing a period is not a concern, you may also experience spotting for two or more cycles which is also normal."

18. Which information does the nurse include when teaching a patient about the use of the norelgestromin-ethinyl estradiol transdermal system (Ortho Evra)? *(Select all that apply.) (626)*
    1. "A new patch should be applied on the same day of the week."
    2. "Contraceptive therapy should be discontinued if pregnancy is confirmed."
    3. "Fold the used patch on itself and flush it down the toilet."
    4. "If the patch is detached for less than 24 hours, apply a new patch to the same location."
    5. "Report serious adverse effects such as severe headache, dizziness, blurred vision, and leg pain as soon as possible."

Discuss osteoporosis and its risk factors as well as preventive measures and the pharmacologic treatment used.

19. A nurse educating a patient about osteoporosis knows further teaching is needed after the patient makes which statement? *(629)*
    1. "So you are saying that with this diagnosis of osteoporosis I will have fragile bones."
    2. "As I understand it, since I am also taking an anticoagulant that it can make the osteoporosis worse."
    3. "If I take more calcium and vitamin D and do strengthening exercises, I can preserve bone strength."
    4. "If I stop smoking and watch my alcohol intake to not exceed two drink daily, I can reverse this osteoporosis."

20. What drugs are used for treatment of osteoporosis? *(Select all that apply.) (629)*
    1. alendronate
    2. denosumab
    3. risedronate
    4. alfuzosin
    5. zoledronic acid

21. The drug class bisphosphonates are used for osteoporosis because they have which drug action? *(630)*
    1. They directly affect the bone reabsorption that occurs by the osteoclasts.
    2. They decrease the rate of bone resorption by inhibiting bone resorption action of the osteoclasts.
    3. They indirectly affect the bone reabsorption rate by enhancing the bone remodeling effect of the osteoblasts.
    4. They cause the calcium and vitamin D in the diet to directly impact the amount of bone laid down for rebuilding.

Describe pharmacologic treatments of benign prostatic hyperplasia.

22. A nurse is describing the difference between the symptoms of obstructive and irritative benign prostatic hyperplasia (BPH) to a patient. Which statement needs to be amended? *(632)*
    1. "The symptoms of irritative BPH include having sudden urinary urgency."
    2. "The symptoms of obstructive BPH include having a reduced urine flow."
    3. "The symptoms of irritative BPH include having a decreased or interrupted urine stream."
    4. "The symptoms of obstructive BPH include having the sensation of incomplete bladder emptying."

23. When teaching a patient about dutasteride (Avodart) therapy for BPH, which statement does the nurse include? *(634)*
    1. "Dutasteride is also used to treat male pattern baldness."
    2. "Dutasteride will cause an increase in serum prostate-specific antigen (PSA) levels."
    3. "If there is no improvement of symptoms after 2 weeks of treatment, the dutasteride will be discontinued."
    4. "Men treated with dutasteride should not donate blood until at least 6 months after stopping therapy."

24. Which medication used for BPH works by inhibiting 5-alpha reductase type 2? *(635)*
    1. finasteride
    2. tamsulosin
    3. dutasteride
    4. sildenafil

Describe the pharmacologic treatment of erectile dysfunction.

25. The nurse is teaching a patient about tadalafil (Cialis) therapy. Which statement made by the patient indicates teaching has been successful? *(636)*
    1. "This drug is an aphrodisiac."
    2. "If I develop chest pain, I will take nitroglycerin."
    3. "I can expect the medication to work within 30 minutes."
    4. "I will take this medication three times a day on a regular basis."

26. Which classification of drugs is used to treat erectile dysfunction? *(636)*
    1. Butyrophenones
    2. Androgen hormone inhibitors
    3. Phosphodiesterase inhibitors
    4. Alpha-1 adrenergic blockers

27. Which statement made by the patient about sildenafil (Viagra) therapy indicates further teaching is needed? *(637-638)*
    1. "I know that Viagra can cause patients to develop glaucoma."
    2. "I know that I should not take nitroglycerin for any angina while I am on Viagra."
    3. "I understand that if I suddenly lose my vision, I need to report it immediately."
    4. "If I get an erection that lasts longer than 4 hours I will seek medical attention."

28. The nurse is educating the patient on the common adverse effects to expect when taking avanafil (Stendra) to treat erectile dysfunction, and includes which statements in the teaching? *(Select all that apply.)* *(637-638)*
    1. "Call your prescriber right away if you develop a sudden loss of vision."
    2. "You need to be careful with nitrates in your food as they will react with the avanafil."
    3. "If you get dizzy or develop low blood pressure, lie down and let the symptoms pass."
    4. "If you develop any headache or flushing in your face and neck, these symptoms tend to be self-limiting."
    5. "It has been reported that if you become color-blind to blue or green, call your prescriber to get a dosage adjustment."

Drugs Used to Treat Disorders of the Urinary System

Answer Key: Textbook page references are provided as a guide for answering these questions. A complete answer key is provided to your instructor.

MATCHING

Match the definition on the right with the key term on the left.

Key Term

1. _____ acidification
2. _____ pyelonephritis
3. _____ frequency
4. _____ urgency
5. _____ overactive bladder syndrome
6. _____ nocturia
7. _____ incontinence

Definition

a. the need to void eight or more times daily
b. waking during the night with the need to void
c. the need to urinate frequently both day and night
d. administering vitamin C to lower the pH of the urine
e. infection of the kidney
f. a compelling desire to urinate that is difficult to ignore
g. the inability to control urine from passing from the bladder

REVIEW QUESTIONS

Scenario: A 52-year-old female patient came to the clinic with complaints of burning on urination and foul-smelling urine. She told the nurse that this happens about twice a year.

Explain the major actions of drugs used to treat disorders of the urinary tract.

8. Which conditions are examples of common urinary tract infections? *(Select all that apply.)* **(640)**
   1. Vaginitis
   2. Cystitis
   3. Pyelonephritis
   4. Urethritis
   5. Prostatitis
9. Which antimicrobial agents are used for bladder infections? *(Select all that apply.)* **(644)**
   1. cephalexin
   2. fosfomycin
   3. linezolid
   4. ciprofloxacin
   5. nitrofurantoin

10. Which statements about phenazopyridine hydro-chloride (Pyridium) for the treatment of patients with urinary tract infections are correct? *(Select all that apply.)* **(649)**
    1. Pyridium reduces bladder spasms.
    2. Pyridium causes the color of urine to become reddish-orange.
    3. Pyridium produces a local anesthetic effect on the mucosa of the ureters and bladder.
    4. Pyridium is most effective against gram-negative bacterial urinary tract infections.
    5. Pyridium relieves burning, pain, urgency, and frequency associated with urinary tract infections.
11. A postpartum patient who had a complicated vaginal delivery of a baby 9 hours ago is unable to void despite multiple nonpharmacologic interventions by the nurse. The nurse expects the healthcare provider to prescribe which drug to facilitate bladder tone and urination? **(649)**
    1. bethanechol chloride (Urecholine)
    2. neostigmine (Prostigmin)
    3. oxybutynin chloride (Ditropan)
    4. tolterodine (Detrol)

12. What is often prescribed to help maintain the acidity of the urine? *(643)*
    1. Vitamin A
    2. Ginkgo biloba
    3. Vitamin C
    4. St. John's wort

13. Which drug acts by interfering with several bacterial enzyme systems? *(644)*
    1. darifenacin (Enablex)
    2. trospium (Sanctura)
    3. mirabegron (Myrbetriq)
    4. nitrofurantoin (Macrodantin)

14. The nurse is teaching the patient in the scenario about which measures that can be taken to prevent the recurrence of urinary tract infections? *(Select all that apply.)* *(643)*
    1. "You only have to take these drugs until your symptoms clear up."
    2. "When you are on these medications for your infection, you will need to drink plenty of fluids."
    3. "It is recommended that you take frequent bubble baths and wear tight underwear."
    4. "It is best to take your antimicrobial agent exactly as prescribed for the entire course of the medication."
    5. "You need to maintain adequate urine volume as a means to treat the overall problem of having recurrent urinary tract infections."

Identify baseline data that the nurse should collect for comparison and evaluation of drug effectiveness.

15. The nurse will assess the patient in the scenario to gather what baseline data? *(Select all that apply.)* *(641)*
    1. History of urinary tract symptoms
    2. Medication history
    3. Nutritional history
    4. History of current symptoms
    5. Obtain a urine sample for analysis

16. What is an important instruction to give patients taking antimicrobial agents for urinary infections? *(643)*
    1. Stop taking the medication when symptoms improve.
    2. Anticipate a skin and sclera discoloration with any antimicrobial agent.
    3. Adequate fluid intake is important because of its effect of diluting the urine.
    4. Symptoms should improve within 5-7 days after taking any antimicrobial agent.

17. Which antimicrobial agent has been approved as a single-dose treatment for urinary tract infections? *(644)*
    1. nitrofurantoin
    2. fosfomycin
    3. mirabegron
    4. oxybutynin

Identify important nursing implementations associated with the drug therapy and treatment of diseases of the urinary system.

18. Which patients are considered to have a urinary tract infection? *(Select all that apply.)* *(640)*
    1. Male with prostatitis
    2. Female with vaginitis
    3. Male with pyelonephritis
    4. Female diagnosed with cystitis
    5. 4-year-old male with urethritis

19. A patient is experiencing burning, frequency, pain, and urgency associated with a urinary tract infection. The nurse expects the healthcare provider to prescribe which medication to treat these symptoms? *(649)*
    1. phenazopyridine hydrochloride (Pyridium)
    2. oxybutynin chloride (Ditropan)
    3. mirabegron (Myrbetriq)
    4. nitrofurantoin (Macrodantin)

20. The nurse knows that an important component of patient education to increase compliance with medications is to determine if the patient can verbalize which points? *(Select all that apply.)* *(643)*
    1. The name of drug
    2. The dosage of the drug
    3. The correct identification of the specific pathogen
    4. The common and adverse effects of the drug
    5. The timing of administration of the drug

21. What important health teaching should the nurse complete for the patient in the scenario? *(Select all that apply.)* *(643)*
    1. Drink plenty of fluids.
    2. Return for urine culture when scheduled.
    3. Continue the medication for the entire course of treatment.
    4. Discuss personal hygiene measures—wiping front to back in females, keeping perineal area clean.
    5. If symptoms such as perineal itching or vaginal discharge occur, wait several days to see if they will resolve on their own.

Identify the symptoms, treatment, and medication used for overactive bladder syndrome.

22. Which statements does the nurse include when teaching a patient about overactive bladder syndrome? *(Select all that apply.)* *(646)*
    1. "You should avoid caffeine."
    2. "Overactive bladder syndrome cannot be cured."
    3. "A chronic infection is the cause of overactive bladder syndrome."
    4. "The first line of pharmacologic treatment of overactive bladder syndrome is anticholinergic agents."
    5. "The goals of therapy for overactive bladder syndrome are to decrease frequency by increasing voided volume, decreasing urgency, and reducing incidents of urinary urge incontinence."

23. Which drugs are included in anticholinergic agents used for overactive bladder syndrome? *(Select all that apply.)* **(647)**
    1. darifenacin (Enablex)
    2. mirabegron (Myrbetriq)
    3. fosfomycin (Monurol)
    4. oxybutynin (Ditropan)
    5. trospium (Sanctura)

24. What are the three primary symptoms of overactive bladder syndrome? **(645)**
    1. Frequency, urinary infections, urinary incontinence
    2. Urgency, nocturia, urge incontinence
    3. Nocturia, frequency, stress incontinence
    4. Frequency, urgency, and urinary incontinence

Drugs Used to Treat Glaucoma and Other Eye Disorders

Answer Key: Textbook page references are provided as a guide for answering these questions. A complete answer key is provided to your instructor.

MATCHING

Match the key term on the right with the definition on the left.

Definition

1. _____ runs radially from the pupillary margin to the iris periphery

2. _____ sudden increase in intraocular pressure (IOP) caused by an obstruction in the iridocorneal angle

3. _____ dilation of the pupils

4. _____ within the iris that encircles the pupil

5. _____ paralysis of the ciliary muscle

6. _____ contraction of the iris sphincter muscle

7. _____ develops insidiously and causes changes in the iridocorneal angle

Key Term

a. miosis
b. mydriasis
c. cycloplegia
d. sphincter muscle
e. open-angle glaucoma
f. closed-angle glaucoma
g. dilator muscle

REVIEW QUESTIONS

Scenario: A 63-year-old male patient comes into the clinic with complaints of pain and constant tearing in his right eye after a flag whipped around his head and caught his eye. He is diagnosed with a corneal abrasion.

Describe the anatomy and physiology of the eye and the normal flow of aqueous humor.

8. What are the layers of the eye? *(Select all that apply.)* *(651)*
   1. Retina
   2. Choroid
   3. Zonular fibers
   4. Corneoscleral coat
   5. Aqueous humor

9. The nurse was educating the patient in the scenario on the anatomy and physiology of the eye. Which statements would be included in the discussion? *(Select all that apply.)* *(651)*
   1. "When the cornea becomes abraded, it is highly susceptible to infection."
   2. "The aqueous humor secretes tears that wash away foreign objects from the eye."
   3. "The cornea is the outermost sheath of the anterior eyeball and is transparent."
   4. "The pupil, or the hole in the iris, is the center black portion of the eye that allows light to reach the retina."
   5. "The lens is a transparent, gelatinous mass of fibers encased in an elastic capsule situated behind the iris."

10. The term *mydriasis* is defined as what? *(651)*
    1. Paralysis of the ciliary muscle
    2. Drainage of aqueous humor out of the eye through drainage channels
    3. Contraction of the iris sphincter muscle, which causes the pupil to narrow
    4. Contraction of the dilator muscle and relaxation of the sphincter muscle, which cause the pupil to dilate

11. How does the eye receive nutrients? *(652)*
    1. Through the aqueous humor
    2. Through the blood vessels
    3. Through the sclera, or the white portion of the eye
    4. Through the thin layer of epithelial cells on the surface of the cornea
12. List in order the flow of aqueous humor in the eye. *(652)*
    1. _____ Flows forward between the lens and the iris into the anterior chamber.
    2. _____ The ciliary body secretes aqueous humor.
    3. _____ Drains out of the eye through drainage channels located near the junction of the cornea and sclera into a meshwork that leads into Schlemm's canal.
    4. _____ It bathes and feeds the lens, the posterior surface of the cornea, and iris.
    5. _____ It flows into the venous system of the eye.
13. When patients have their IOP measured, it determines the eye's what? *(653)*
    1. Tear duct capacity
    2. Resistance from the ciliary bodies
    3. Amount of aqueous humor
    4. Ability to contract and relax the dilator muscle

Identify the changes in normal flow of aqueous humor caused by open-angle and closed-angle glaucoma.

14. What happens when patients have open-angle glaucoma? *(653)*
    1. The posterior chamber narrows, causing an increase in IOP.
    2. The anterior chamber overflows into the posterior chamber, causing an increase in IOP.
    3. The sudden increase in IOP is caused by a mechanical obstruction in the iridocorneal angle.
    4. IOP is gradually increased because of the changes in the iridocorneal angle that prevent the outflow of aqueous humor.
15. The nurse was discussing the difference between open-angle glaucoma and closed-angle glaucoma with a patient who was newly diagnosed with glaucoma. Which statement by the patient indicates more teaching is needed? *(653)*
    1. "Closed-angle glaucoma is the one that suddenly develops."
    2. "Open-angle glaucoma is the kind that develops slowly."
    3. "Glaucoma can be cured by taking eyedrops for 2 weeks."
    4. "Glaucoma is an eye disorder that develops because the pressure inside your eyeball is too high."

16. Of the three types of glaucoma, which one requires surgical intervention to correct? *(653)*
    1. Primary
    2. Secondary
    3. Tertiary
    4. Congenital

Explain patient assessments needed for eye disorders.

17. What is typically included in an eye exam that the nurse performs for the patient in the scenario with an eye injury? *(Select all that apply.)* *(654)*
    1. Check for eyelid edema.
    2. Observe for and report nystagmus.
    3. Observe for any redness or drainage of the eyes.
    4. Ask whether there is any history of colorblindness.
    5. Ask whether glasses or contact lenses are worn.
18. One of the greatest challenges in the care of chronic eye disorders such as glaucoma is convincing the patient of what? *(656)*
    1. The need to wear an eye patch every night to prevent eye strain
    2. The importance of not taking any over-the-counter or herbal products
    3. The differences among cataracts, glaucoma, and macular degeneration
    4. The need for long-term treatment and adherence to the therapeutic regimen
19. What common adverse effect will the nurse assess in patients who are receiving cholinergic agents? *(658)*
    1. Bleeding tendencies
    2. Circulatory overload symptoms
    3. Reduced visual acuity especially at night
    4. Allergies to sulfonamide antibiotics

Review the correct procedure for instilling eyedrops or eye ointments and discuss patient teaching needs for glaucoma medication use.

20. List in the correct order how to instill eyedrops or eye ointment. *(656)*
    1. _____ Perform hand hygiene and don gloves.
    2. _____ Approach the eye from below.
    3. _____ Apply gentle pressure using a clean tissue to the inner canthus of the eyelid.
    4. _____ Instruct the patient to look up, and instill drops or squeeze ointment into the conjunctival sac.
    5. _____ Expose the lower conjunctival sac by applying gentle traction.

21. Which statements does the nurse include when teaching a patient about health promotion after eye surgery? *(Select all that apply.)* *(656)*
    1. "Avoid bending at the waist."
    2. "Avoid any straining with stool."
    3. "Cough at least 10 times every hour."
    4. "Report any pain not relieved by prescribed medications."
    5. "Use aseptic technique when instilling eye medications."

22. To prevent systemic effects of ophthalmic cholinergic agents, the nurse carefully blocks the inner canthus of the eye for how many minutes? *(656)*
    1. 1-2
    2. 3-5
    3. 8-10
    4. 12-14

23. What are systemic adverse effects of the anticholinergic agent atropine sulfate? *(Select all that apply.)* *(662)*
    1. Bradycardia
    2. Diarrhea
    3. Blurred vision
    4. Vasodilation
    5. Dry mouth

24. What mechanism of action do carbonic anhydrase inhibitors have on the eye? *(656)*
    1. They increase tearing and widen the nasolacrimal ducts.
    2. They widen the filtration angle, permitting an outflow of aqueous humor.
    3. They decrease the flow of aqueous humor by closing the iridocorneal angle.
    4. They inhibit the enzyme carbonic anhydrase, which results in a decrease in aqueous humor production.

25. Cholinergic agents produce contraction of the iris (miosis) and ciliary body musculature (accommodation), by which mechanism of action? *(658)*
    1. They absorb acetylcholine at nerve synapses.
    2. They cause vasoconstriction of the blood vessels in the eye.
    3. Their effect results in a reduced production of aqueous humor.
    4. They cause a widening of the filtration angle, thus decreasing IOP.

26. Adrenergic agents have several mechanisms of action, including what? *(Select all that apply.)* *(659-660)*
    1. They cause the pupil to dilate and relax the ciliary muscle.
    2. They cause a decrease in the formation of aqueous humor.
    3. They cause an increase in the outflow of aqueous humor.
    4. They cause vasoconstriction of the blood vessels in the eye.
    5. They cause the absorption of an excess volume of aqueous humor.

27. How are beta-adrenergic blocking agents thought to work when given for the treatment of glaucoma? *(660)*
    1. By reducing the production of aqueous humor
    2. By increasing the filtration angle, thus decreasing IOP
    3. By absorbing the excess volume of aqueous humor
    4. By inhibiting any cholinergic activity within the eye

28. What mechanism of action do prostaglandin agonists have on the eye? *(660)*
    1. They absorb aqueous humor.
    2. They reduce the production of aqueous humor.
    3. They reduce IOP by increasing the outflow of aqueous humor.
    4. They cause vasoconstriction of the blood vessels in the eye.

Drugs Used to Treat Cancer

Answer Key: Textbook page references are provided as a guide for answering these questions. A complete answer key is provided to your instructor.

MATCHING
Match the definition on the left with the term on the right.

Definition

1. _____ biologic therapies that include cytokines, monoclonal antibodies, growth factors, and vaccines

2. _____ chemotherapy that uses cell cycle–specific and cell cycle–nonspecific agents

3. _____ meaning new growth; can refer to benign or malignant cells

4. _____ abnormal cell growth that invades surrounding tissues and develops growths in other tissues distant to the site of origin

5. _____ agents that help reduce the toxicity of chemotherapeutic agents to normal cells

6. _____ cancer cells that metastasize to other organs of the body

Term

a. metastases
b. malignant
c. targeted anticancer agents
d. chemoprotective agents
e. neoplastic disease
f. combination therapy

REVIEW QUESTIONS

Scenario: A 48-year-old woman, mother of three, was newly diagnosed with breast cancer and was very distraught in the outpatient clinic when she came for her first chemotherapy treatment.

Cite the goals of chemotherapy.

7. What are the goals of chemotherapy? *(Select all that apply.) (669)*
   1. Control growth of the cancer cells
   2. Long-term survival or a cure of cancer
   3. Use phase-nonspecific chemotherapy agents exclusively
   4. Give when new pathways of tumor cell metabolism are discovered
   5. Give doses large enough to kill the cancer cells but small enough for normal cells to live

8. After educating the patient in the scenario about the best timing for giving chemotherapy, the nurse knows that which statement by the patient would indicate further teaching is needed? *(676)*
   1. "I know that the overall goal of chemotherapy in general is to give enough drug to kill the cancer without too much damage to the normal cells."
   2. "I understand it is important to deliver the chemotherapy at precise intervals to impact the cancer cells' growth cycle."
   3. "I can prevent complications from the chemotherapy through proper diet and hygiene."
   4. "I understand that when I am on chemotherapy, I can have fresh flowers as long as I do not touch them and I can eat fresh vegetables that I wash thoroughly."

9. For the patient and family to manage the chemotherapy treatment regimen, an understanding of which points needs to be stressed? *(Select all that apply.) (677)*
   1. Name of the drug
   2. Right documentation
   3. Common and serious adverse effects
   4. Time of administration
   5. Dosage and route of the drug

10. Treatment of cancer often requires multiple different approaches, which may include what modalities? *(Select all that apply.)* **(668)**
    1. Surgery
    2. Radiation
    3. Biologic therapies
    4. Targeted drug therapy
    5. Phlebotomy

Describe the role of targeted anticancer agents in treating cancer.

11. What does the choice of chemotherapeutic agents used to help fight cancer depend on? *(Select all that apply.)* **(670)**
    1. The size of the tumor
    2. The type of tumor cell
    3. The potency of the agent
    4. The rate of growth of the cancer
    5. The frequency of the agents' administration

12. What is the role of targeted anticancer agents in treating cancer? **(671)**
    1. They trigger the recovery of the bone marrow cells.
    2. They cause cell death by means that are unknown.
    3. They reduce the toxic effects of the chemotherapy agents.
    4. They act on receptors that are specific to the cancer cells' growth factors.

13. Which classifications of drugs are considered part of the traditional major groups of chemotherapeutic agents? *(Select all that apply.)* **(670)**
    1. Hormones
    2. Antimetabolites
    3. Natural products
    4. Prostaglandin inhibitors
    5. Antineoplastic antibiotics

14. Which are biologic therapies or targeted anticancer agents? *(Select all that apply.)* **(671)**
    1. Cytokines
    2. Vaccines
    3. Growth factors
    4. Monoclonal antibodies
    5. Cholinesterase inhibitors

Identify how chemoprotective agents are used in treating cancer.

15. The reason chemoprotective agents are used to treat cancer is because they will have what effect? **(671)**
    1. They stimulate red blood cell production.
    2. They target the cancer cells specifically.
    3. They trigger the recovery of bone marrow cells.
    4. They reduce the toxic effects of the chemotherapy agents on normal cells.

16. Which medications are used as chemoprotective agents? *(Select all that apply.)* **(671)**
    1. sargramostim (Leukine)
    2. mesna (Mesnex)
    3. dexrazoxane (Zinecard)
    4. amifostine (Ethyol)
    5. filgrastim (Neupogen)

17. The nurse was explaining to the patient in the scenario the reason for the medication Zinecard that she was receiving after her chemotherapy. Which statement by the patient indicates further teaching is needed? **(671)**
    1. "I understand that Zinecard is to reduce the chances of developing cardiomyopathy from the doxorubicin I'm taking."
    2. "The drug Zinecard will stimulate my bone marrow to produce red blood cells."
    3. "Because I am taking Zinecard, I should be able to take the full therapeutic dose of chemotherapy."
    4. "As I understand it, this drug Zinecard is designed to reduce the toxic effects of my chemotherapy."

18. The nurse is administering a chemotherapeutic agent and knows which precautions must be observed for safe handling of these agents? *(Select all that apply.)* **(672)**
    1. Prevent any inhalation of aerosols.
    2. Carefully mix the agents in the med room.
    3. Prevent contamination of body fluids.
    4. Expect that the route of the agents depends on the cancer.
    5. Prevent any drug absorption through the skin.

Discuss bone marrow stimulants and their effect and use.

19. What do the bone marrow stimulants do in the treatment of cancer? **(672)**
    1. They induce anemia.
    2. They stimulate the resting phase of the cell.
    3. They trigger an increase of killer T cells.
    4. They trigger the recovery of bone marrow cells.

20. The nurse anticipates the use of which medication to treat a patient with chemotherapy-induced anemia by stimulating the production of RBCs? **(672)**
    1. sargramostim (Leukine)
    2. glucarpidase (Voraxaze)
    3. epoetin alfa (Epogen)
    4. filgrastim (Neupogen)

21. In which situation would the use of bone marrow stimulants be appropriate? *(Select all that apply.)* **(672)**
    1. When treating leukemia
    2. During lymphoma therapy
    3. During bone marrow transplantation
    4. To control cell membrane receptor response
    5. To reduce the toxic effects of chemotherapy

22. Use of bone marrow stimulants to allow the immune system to recover earlier than would occur naturally results in what major benefit? *(672)*
    1. Preventing chronic renal failure
    2. Stopping infections from becoming pathologic
    3. Allowing the patient to have fewer cycles of chemotherapy
    4. Delaying the effects of anticipated nausea and vomiting

Describe the nursing assessments and interventions needed to help alleviate the adverse effects of chemotherapy.

23. Which are baseline assessments by the nurse for the patient in the scenario that are needed during the initiation of cancer therapy? *(Select all that apply.)* *(672-673)*
    1. Determine the exposure to tobacco and tobacco smoke.
    2. Identify the usual eating and elimination patterns.
    3. Ask about the understanding the patient has of the diagnosis.
    4. Review the medication history for any drugs that may have caused cancer.
    5. Ask about a history of viral disease that may have caused cancer.

24. Which adverse effects from chemotherapy does the nurse monitor patients for? *(Select all that apply.)* *(674-675)*
    1. Stomatitis
    2. Infection
    3. Heat intolerance
    4. Changes in bowel patterns
    5. Nausea and vomiting

25. A patient has severe lesions in his mouth as an adverse effect of chemotherapy. When does the nurse suggest the patient perform oral hygiene measures using prescribed local anesthetic and antimicrobial solutions? *(675)*
    1. After each meal
    2. Once every 8 hours
    3. Hourly while the patient is awake
    4. In the morning when the patient awakens and before bed

26. Cancer care that applies to all patients includes which interventions? *(Select all that apply.)* *(673)*
    1. Allowing rest periods
    2. Determining activity tolerance
    3. Attending to pain management
    4. Anticipating that diarrhea will occur
    5. Limiting the amount of self-care allowed

Drugs Used to Treat the Musculoskeletal System

44

Answer Key: Textbook page references are provided as a guide for answering these questions. A complete answer key is provided to your instructor.

MATCHING

Match the definition on the right to the key term on the left.

Key Term

1. _____ cerebral palsy
2. _____ multiple sclerosis
3. _____ stroke syndrome
4. _____ hypercapnia
5. _____ spasticity
6. _____ muscle spasms
7. _____ gout

Definition

a. an upper motor neuron disorder characterized by muscle hypertonicity and involuntary jerks
b. caused by an injury or birth defect, characterized by exaggerated reflexes, abnormal posture, involuntary movements, and difficulty walking
c. elevated carbon dioxide levels causing tachycardia, hypotension, and cyanosis
d. sudden alternating contractions and relaxations or sustained contractions of muscle
e. a common and treatable form of inflammatory arthritis
f. an autoimmune disease affecting the brain and spinal cord
g. caused by an embolism, thrombosis, or ruptured aneurysm; characteristics include a sudden onset of vertigo, numbness, aphasia, and dysarthria, along with hemiplegia

REVIEW QUESTIONS

Scenario: A 35-year-old male patient with cerebral palsy came into the outpatient clinic because he was scheduled to have his baclofen pump refilled.

Describe the nursing assessment data needed to evaluate a patient with a skeletal muscle disorder.

8. The nurse will need to obtain a medication history from the patient in the scenario, and asks which appropriate questions? *(Select all that apply.) (680)*
   1. "Do you use any assistive devices?"
   2. "What is the extent of your usual daily exercise?"
   3. "What medications did you take today and when?"
   4. "Do you use any nonpharmacologic treatments like a heating pad or acupuncture?"
   5. "Do you have a list of all the prescribed and over-the-counter medications that you are taking?"

9. A 32-year-old man came to the outpatient clinic complaining about a recent injury sustained while jogging and subsequent left knee pain. The nurse knows further education is needed after the patient makes which statement? *(681)*
   1. "I can put ice on my knee to help with the swelling for 48 hours."
   2. "I will have to elevate my leg initially to reduce swelling and pain."
   3. "I can immobilize my knee with an elastic wrap to help with the pain."
   4. "I can use hot packs on my knee initially to help with the pain."

10. The nurse needs to gather important assessment data on the patient in the scenario including what factors? *(Select all that apply.) (680)*
    1. Assessing the mental status of the patient
    2. Determining the degree of respiratory depression
    3. Evaluating the capillary refill and any presence of paresthesias
    4. Noting any differences in circumference, symmetry, or length of limbs
    5. Assessing muscle strength by asking the patient to lift his head off the pillow

Identify the therapeutic response and the common and serious adverse effects from skeletal muscle relaxant therapy.

11. What is the mechanism of action for the centrally acting skeletal muscle relaxants? *(682)*
    1. They directly affect the muscles.
    2. They cause CNS depression.
    3. They affect nerve conduction.
    4. They cause the neuromuscular junctions to be desensitized to stimuli.

12. Which statement by a patient taking dantrolene (Dantrium) for treatment of muscle spasticity of stroke syndrome indicates that more patient education is needed? *(685)*
    1. "I will avoid exposure to the sun, but I can still use a tanning lamp."
    2. "I will notify my healthcare provider if my skin turns yellow."
    3. "I know that it might take up to a week for me to see any response to this drug."
    4. "If I develop adverse effects from this medication, I will not discontinue treatment until I notify my healthcare provider."

13. For which adverse effects does the nurse need to evaluate the patient in the scenario, related to the baclofen pump? *(Select all that apply.) (684)*
    1. Drowsiness
    2. Fatigue
    3. Headache
    4. Back pain
    5. Dizziness

Describe the effect of centrally acting skeletal muscle relaxants on the central nervous system (CNS) and the safety precautions required during their use.

14. Which statements about centrally acting skeletal muscle relaxants are true? *(Select all that apply.) (682)*
    1. They produce sedation in patients receiving them.
    2. They have a direct effect on the neuromuscular junction, causing relaxation.
    3. They produce their therapeutic effect by depressing the central nervous system.
    4. They directly relax the muscles by suppressing nerve conduction at the neuromuscular junction.
    5. They are the agents of choice for the treatment of muscle spasticity associated with cerebral or spinal cord disease.

15. The nurse was reviewing which laboratory results to determine if the patient on chlorzoxazone (Lorzone) was exhibiting any hepatotoxicity? *(Select all that apply.) (683)*
    1. GGT
    2. WBC
    3. RBC
    4. AST
    5. ALT

16. Which medications are considered centrally acting skeletal muscle relaxants? *(Select all that apply.) (683)*
    1. metaxalone (Skelaxin)
    2. dantrolene (Dantrium)
    3. cyclobenzaprine (Amrix)
    4. allopurinol (Zyloprim)
    5. carisoprodol (Soma)

Describe the physiologic effects of neuromuscular blocking agents and assessments needed, as well as the equipment needed in the immediate patient care area when neuromuscular blocking agents are administered.

17. Which are examples of when it would be appropriate to use neuromuscular blocking agents? *(Select all that apply.) (681)*
    1. When patients have tetanus
    2. When patients develop nystagmus
    3. During the administration of general anesthesia
    4. When intubating patients and preventing laryngospasm
    5. During the administration of electroshock therapy to prevent muscular activity

18. Why would patients with myasthenia gravis, spinal cord injuries, or multiple sclerosis need to be carefully identified prior to administration of neuromuscular blocking agents? *(686)*
    1. Postoperatively, they will experience respiratory depression for a prolonged period.
    2. They will develop the adverse effect of histamine release much faster than other patients.
    3. They will require larger doses of the agents to get the same effect as other patients.
    4. They need careful adjustments in dosages to assess their ability to tolerate the agents.

19. Which drugs are antidotes for neuromuscular blocking agents? *(Select all that apply.) (685)*
    1. naloxone
    2. pyridostigmine bromide
    3. edrophonium chloride
    4. neostigmine methylsulfate
    5. ethacrynic acid

20. A patient who has returned from abdominal surgery reports pain. The patient had received a neuromuscular blocking agent as part of the anesthesia for the surgery. What additional information is essential for the nurse to obtain before administering the prescribed analgesic? *(686)*
    1. Respirations
    2. Family history
    3. Estimated time of discharge
    4. Laboratory results for CBC and electrolytes

21. Which description of patients receiving neuromuscular blocking agents is accurate? *(686)*
    1. They experience complete analgesia.
    2. They have an enhanced cough reflex.
    3. They experience a decrease in salivation.
    4. They are at risk for the development of bronchospasm, edema, and urticaria.

22. Which statements about the effects of neuromuscular blocking agents in patients with muscular disorders are true? *(Select all that apply.)* *(685)*
    1. Neuromuscular blocking agents have no effect on memory.
    2. Neuromuscular blocking agents have no effect on consciousness.
    3. Neuromuscular blocking agents have no effect on pain threshold.
    4. The IV route is the only method for administering neuromuscular blocking agents.
    5. Pain medications are contraindicated in patients receiving neuromuscular blocking agents.

Describe the nursing assessment data needed to evaluate a patient with gout.

23. The nurse is preparing to administer colchicine for a patient with gout and needs to assess the patient for what? *(Select all that apply.)* *(687)*
    1. Current bowel status
    2. Ability to cough and swallow adequately
    3. Laboratory values for uric acid, BUN, and AST
    4. Degree of spasticity involving the affected limb
    5. Level and location of pain, using the pain rating scale

24. After completing the education for the patient in the scenario on the use of colchicine, the nurse will need to provide further education when the patient makes which statement? *(687)*
    1. "I need to take this to prevent an attack of gout."
    2. "My joint swelling will subside within 12 hours."
    3. "It will take from 48-72 hours before I will get any pain relief."
    4. "I know I can take a dose every 3 days to prevent an attack of gout."

25. How does probenecid prevent acute attacks of gouty arthritis? *(687)*
    1. It dissolves uric acid crystals.
    2. It inhibits the production of uric acid.
    3. It relieves the pain in joints affected by gout.
    4. It enhances the excretion of uric acid by the kidneys.

Identify the therapeutic response and the common and serious adverse effects from gout medications.

26. What is the primary therapeutic outcome of colchicine therapy? *(687)*
    1. Dissolve uric acid crystals
    2. Inhibit the production of uric acid
    3. Decrease the amount of uric acid in the blood or urine
    4. Eliminate joint pain secondary to acute gout attack

27. The nurse has provided patient teaching for probenecid therapy. Which statement by the patient indicates that more teaching is needed? *(687)*
    1. "This drug works on the tissues of my great toe, where I usually get the gout, to get rid of the problem."
    2. "I can expect that the incidence of gout attacks may increase for the first few months of therapy with this drug."
    3. "I will tell my healthcare provider if I develop vomiting that looks like coffee grounds."
    4. "If I develop a rash, I will tell my healthcare provider because this most likely means that I have an allergy to this drug."

28. The nurse knows that bone marrow depression can occur as an adverse effect with xanthine oxidase inhibitors and will monitor for which effects? *(Select all that apply.)* *(689)*
    1. Sore throat
    2. Restlessness
    3. Jaundice
    4. Progressive weakness
    5. Cardiac arrhythmias

Antimicrobial Agents

Answer Key: Textbook page references are provided as a guide for answering these questions. A complete answer key is provided to your instructor.

MATCHING
Match the definition on the left with the term on the right.

Definition

1. _____ examples include: *Acinetobacter spp., Providencia spp., Escherichia coli*, and *Klebsiella spp.*

2. _____ damage to the eighth cranial nerve, causing dizziness, tinnitus, and hearing loss

3. _____ microorganisms that are toxic to patients

4. _____ examples include: *Staphylococcus aureus, S. epidermidis, Streptococcus pyogenes*, and *S. pneumoniae*

5. _____ antimicrobial therapy given to patients at risk for developing infections

6. _____ damage to the kidney, causing increased creatinine and BUN, and decreased urine output

7. _____ reduced circulating prothrombin, with and without bleeding

Term

a. pathogenic
b. prophylactic antibiotics
c. nephrotoxicity
d. ototoxicity
e. hypoprothrombinemia
f. gram-negative microorganisms
g. gram-positive microorganisms

REVIEW QUESTIONS

Scenario: An 89-year-old male patient was admitted to the hospital with urosepsis. He has a history of diabetes, hypertension, hypothyroidism, depression, functional decline, and gastroesophageal reflux disease (GERD).

Explain the major actions and effects of classes of drugs used to treat infectious diseases.

8. Antibiotics from the drug class macrolides have which action on bacteria? *(704)*
   1. They prevent the bacteria from making folic acid.
   2. They inhibit the ability of the bacteria to synthesize protein.
   3. They inhibit the ability of the bacteria to create a cell wall.
   4. They weaken the cell wall of the bacteria so that the contents spill out.

9. Which conditions would aminoglycosides be used to treat? *(Select all that apply.) (696)*
   1. Wound infections
   2. Latent tuberculosis
   3. Viral infections
   4. Life-threatening septicemia
   5. Gram-negative bacteria causing meningitis

10. The antimicrobial agents from the drug class carbapenems act on bacteria by what mechanism of action? *(698)*
    1. They inhibit cell membrane synthesis.
    2. They prevent bacteria from making folic acid.
    3. They inhibit the ability of the bacteria to create a cell wall.
    4. They weaken the cell wall of the bacteria so that the contents spill out.

11. What is the mechanism of action of the class of antibiotics known as streptogramins? *(711)*
    1. They destroy the bacterial cell wall.
    2. They interfere with bacterial DNA.
    3. They inhibit protein synthesis in bacterial cells.
    4. They inhibit the bacteria's ability to make folic acid.

12. Which class of antimicrobials is chemically related to penicillin and acts by inhibiting cell wall synthesis? *(700)*
    1. Quinolones
    2. Macrolides
    3. Streptogramins
    4. Cephalosporins
13. Which statement best describes the mechanism of action of the quinolones? *(709)*
    1. They destroy the bacterial cell wall.
    2. They inhibit the activity of DNA gyrase.
    3. They inhibit protein synthesis in bacterial cells.
    4. They inhibit the bacteria's ability to make folic acid.
14. What is the mechanism of action of amphotericin B? *(723)*
    1. Inhibiting biosynthesis of folic acid
    2. Inhibiting DNA synthesis of the cells
    3. Disruption of the cell membrane of fungal cells
    4. Interfering with the enzyme needed for cell wall generation
15. Which class of antimicrobials is reserved for serious life-threatening infections that are vancomycin-resistant, and act by inhibiting protein synthesis in bacterial cells? *(711)*
    1. Carbapenems
    2. Streptogramins
    3. Quinolones
    4. Cephalosporins
16. Which antibiotic is effective against aerobic and anaerobic bacteria, and acts by inhibiting bacterial cell wall synthesis? *(698)*
    1. levofloxacin
    2. sulfadiazine
    3. ertapenem
    4. gentamicin

List the signs and symptoms of a secondary infection.
17. The nurse will monitor the patient in the scenario carefully for which signs and symptoms of a secondary infection? *(Select all that apply.) (694)*
    1. Anal lesions
    2. Severe diarrhea
    3. Phlebitis at the IV site
    4. Tinnitus and progressive hearing loss
    5. White patches in the oral cavity
18. Which measures may be taken by the nurse to minimize the effects of a secondary infection? *(Select all that apply.) (694)*
    1. Practice good personal hygiene.
    2. Hold the prescribed antimicrobial medication when effects are noticed.
    3. Monitor for the development of symptoms of secondary infection.
    4. Administer additional antimicrobials effective against the new organism.
    5. Notify the healthcare provider if signs and symptoms of a secondary infection occur.

19. After completing education on tigecycline therapy for the patient in the scenario, the nurse knows that more teaching is needed when the patient makes which statement? *(704)*
    1. "I know I need adequate rest and as little stress as possible."
    2. "If I develop any diarrhea, I will just take some over-the-counter Lomotil."
    3. "I know that my kidneys may be affected with this antibiotic, so I will report any decline in my urine output."
    4. "If I notice any symptoms like sore throat, bruising, or worsening fatigue, I need to report them immediately."
20. Which symptoms of hepatotoxicity will the patient be able to monitor for after discharge from the hospital? *(Select all that apply.) (694)*
    1. Anorexia
    2. Jaundice
    3. Elevated creatinine
    4. Hepatomegaly
    5. Nausea and vomiting
21. A patient newly prescribed the cephalosporin Ceclor asked the nurse how she would know if she was experiencing an allergic reaction. What would be an appropriate response by the nurse? *(694)*
    1. "Most of the time it will just be a rash on your arm."
    2. "The drug Ceclor does not have any allergies associated with it."
    3. "Nausea, vomiting, and diarrhea are the most common symptoms of an allergic reaction."
    4. "Trouble breathing, skin rashes, or facial edema may be symptoms of an allergic reaction."

Describe the signs and symptoms of the common adverse effects of antimicrobial therapy.
22. What are the "big three" common adverse effects associated with antimicrobial therapy? *(Select all that apply.) (694)*
    1. Nausea
    2. Vomiting
    3. Allergies
    4. Constipation
    5. Diarrhea
23. The patient in the scenario was started on cefuroxime for his infection. Which medication prescribed for another clinical condition did the nurse notice was contraindicated with cefuroxime, requiring notifying the prescriber? *(702)*
    1. metformin (Glucophage)
    2. atenolol (Tenormin)
    3. famotidine (Pepcid)
    4. levothyroxine (Synthroid)

24. A patient who was being treated for cellulitis returned to the clinic with complaints of his arm looking sunburnt and developing patches that itch after being outside. The nurse recognizes these symptoms as what? *(695)*
    1. Blood dyscrasia
    2. Photosensitivity
    3. Nephrotoxicity
    4. Secondary infection

Describe the nursing assessments and interventions for the common adverse effects associated with antimicrobial agents: allergic reaction, nephrotoxicity, ototoxicity, and hepatotoxicity.

25. The severe adverse reaction of nephrotoxicity from antimicrobial therapy can be monitored by which laboratory results? *(Select all that apply.)* *(694)*
    1. AST
    2. Creatinine
    3. WBC
    4. BUN
    5. Hgb

26. Prior to administration of a carbapenem, what premedication assessments should the nurse perform? *(Select all that apply.)* *(698)*
    1. Check hydration status.
    2. Check vital signs.
    3. Assess basic mental status.
    4. Check any allergies specifically to penicillin and cephalosporins.
    5. Determine that the organism being treated is *Candida albicans.*

27. The nurse was performing a premedication assessment before therapy with cephalosporins on a patient. Which condition observed in the patient would indicate the drug should be held and the healthcare provider notified? *(700)*
    1. Exophthalmos
    2. Oral candidiasis
    3. Onychomycosis of the toenail
    4. Low urine output and concentrated urine

28. Which antimicrobial agent would be contraindicated in a patient who will be receiving neuromuscular blockade for a surgical procedure? *(697)*
    1. Sulfonamides (i.e., sulfadiazine)
    2. Quinolones (i.e., norfloxacin)
    3. Aminoglycosides (i.e., neomycin)
    4. Carbapenems (i.e., ertapenem)

29. Why is it essential to report the occurrence of severe diarrhea with antibiotic therapy? *(694)*
    1. This would indicate nephrotoxicity.
    2. This may mean that the drug is not being absorbed any further.
    3. This may indicate drug-induced pseudomembranous colitis.
    4. This would indicate that an allergic response has occurred.

30. The assessment data that the nurse will monitor for the patient in the scenario who has now been receiving antibiotics for his infection, include noting which signs and symptoms? *(Select all that apply.)* *(694)*
    1. Any photosensitivity
    2. Any allergic reactions
    3. When his last vaccination for flu was given
    4. Changes in laboratory results (i.e., BUN and creatinine)
    5. Any symptoms that may indicate a secondary infection is developing

31. When administering aminoglycosides to a patient, what does the nurse assess? *(Select all that apply.)* *(697)*
    1. Any history of renal disease
    2. Adequate hydration status related to any nausea and vomiting
    3. Any development of dizziness, tinnitus, and progressive hearing loss
    4. Whether anesthesia was administered to the patient within the past 48-72 hours
    5. Any allergy to penicillin because patients allergic to penicillin are allergic to aminoglycosides

Cite the primary uses for antibiotic agents, antitubercular agents, antifungal agents, and antiviral agents.

32. Antimicrobial agents can be classified according to which types of pathogenic organism? *(Select all that apply.)* *(692)*
    1. Pollen
    2. Fungus
    3. Cerumen
    4. Viruses
    5. Bacteria

33. The therapeutic outcome expected from tigecycline (Tygacil) is elimination of bacterial infection, and should be used when? *(704)*
    1. Against viruses
    2. As a bacteriostatic antibiotic
    3. In children and adolescents
    4. The pathogen is resistant to other available antibiotics

34. Which infections can macrolides be used for? *(Select all that apply.)* *(705)*
    1. Respiratory
    2. Gastrointestinal tract
    3. Prophylactic before surgery
    4. Sexually transmitted infection
    5. Skin and soft-tissue infections

35. Which are clinical uses of penicillins? *(Select all that apply.)* *(708)*
    1. Treatment of pneumonia
    2. Treatment of middle-ear infection
    3. Treatment of urinary tract infections
    4. Prophylactic antibiotic for meningitis
    5. Prophylactic antibiotic for syphilis and gonorrhea

36. Because the sulfonamides inhibit bacterial biosynthesis of folic acid, which laboratory value needs to be monitored periodically when patients are on these antibiotics? *(713)*
    1. Electrolytes
    2. PT and platelets
    3. Creatinine and BUN
    4. CBC with differential

37. What are the effects of administering tetracyclines during pregnancy? *(713)*
    1. They may cause dental caries.
    2. They may cause tooth enamel staining.
    3. They may cause birth defects.
    4. They may cause preterm labor.

38. The nurse preparing isoniazid and rifampin to be administered to a patient knows that these antibiotics are being given for the treatment of what? *(716-717)*
    1. Syphilis
    2. Trichinosis
    3. Tuberculosis
    4. Cellulitis

39. What is the topical antifungal agent ketoconazole used to treat? *(Select all that apply.)* *(724)*
    1. Histoplasmosis
    2. Tinea pedis (athlete's foot)
    3. Candidiasis (thrush)
    4. Cutaneous candidiasis (diaper rash)
    5. Cryptococcal meningitis

Nutrition

Answer Key: Textbook page references are provided as a guide for answering these questions. A complete answer key is provided to your instructor.

MATCHING
Match the definition on the right with the key term on the left.

Key Term

1. _____ Dietary Reference Intakes (DRIs)
2. _____ Estimated Average Requirement (EAR)
3. _____ Recommended Dietary Allowances (RDAs)
4. _____ Adequate Intake (AI)
5. _____ Tolerable Upper Intake Level (UL)
6. _____ Estimated Energy Requirement (EER)
7. _____ marasmus
8. _____ kwashiorkor

Definition

a. the highest level of daily nutrient intake that is likely to pose no risk of adverse health effects
b. a list of average daily dietary intake level that meets the nutrient requirements of almost all healthy individuals in a group
c. the most common form of malnutrition in hospitalized patients
d. the average dietary energy intake that is predicted to maintain energy balance in healthy adults
e. provides quantitative estimates of nutrient intakes for planning and assessing diets
f. a protein deficiency that develops when little or no protein is in the diet
g. a nutrient intake value that is estimated to meet the requirement of half of the healthy individuals in a group
h. a value based on observed or experimentally determined approximations of nutrient intake by a group of healthy people

REVIEW QUESTIONS

Scenario: A 75-year-old female patient came to the clinic with complaints of fatigue and increasing weakness. She has been losing weight, has poor appetite, and noticed that her hair is dry and falls out easily.

Identify sources of dietary fiber and dietary fats.

9. What are the essential macronutrients needed by the body? *(Select all that apply.)* **(736)**
   1. Fats
   2. Fiber
   3. Water
   4. Proteins
   5. Carbohydrates

10. The nurse educating a patient on his diet with regards to the recommended primary sources of fats, suggested which fat sources are healthy? *(Select all that apply.)* **(739)**
    1. Coconut oil
    2. Olive oil
    3. Peanut oil
    4. Avocados
    5. Soybean oil

11. Which fat source is of concern because it has no known nutritional benefit? **(737)**
    1. Trans fats
    2. Saturated fats
    3. Polyunsaturated fats
    4. Monounsaturated fats

12. The *2015-2020 Dietary Guidelines for Americans* has recommended dietary patterns that are rich in what? *(Select all that apply.)* *(737-738)*
    1. Vegetables
    2. Ice cream
    3. Legumes
    4. Seafood
    5. Whole grains

Differentiate between fat-soluble and water-soluble vitamins and discuss their functions.

13. Which vitamins are considered water-soluble? *(Select all that apply.)* *(744)*
    1. Niacin
    2. Retinol
    3. Ascorbic acid
    4. Cyanocobalamin
    5. Phytonadione

14. The nurse was administering cholecalciferol to a patient who asks what it is. What is an appropriate response by the nurse? *(744)*
    1. "I believe this is vitamin E."
    2. "This is another name for vitamin B."
    3. "It is one of those water-soluble vitamins that are necessary in your diet."
    4. "This is vitamin D, which helps regulate calcium and phosphorus metabolism."

15. The nurse discussing with a patient the foods that contain vitamin B_2 will provide further teaching after the patient makes which statement? *(744)*
    1. "Another name for vitamin B_2 is riboflavin."
    2. "I can get vitamin B_2 in my diet by eating pork, peas, and dry beans."
    3. "If I eat green leafy vegetables, fruit, and eggs, I will being getting some vitamin B_2."
    4. "I know that vitamin B_2 is important because it is needed for normal cell function."

Discuss the functions of minerals in the body.

16. Which mineral found in iodized salt and seafood is a component of thyroid hormones? *(745)*
    1. Chromium
    2. Chlorine
    3. Fluorine
    4. Iodine

17. Which mineral found in grains, green leafy vegetables, nuts, and legumes is essential for protein synthesis and nerve transmission? *(745)*
    1. Magnesium
    2. Manganese
    3. Phosphorus
    4. Chromium

18. Which mineral found in whole grains, cereals, green vegetables, and tea is essential for fat and connective tissue synthesis? *(745)*
    1. Calcium
    2. Manganese
    3. Magnesium
    4. Cobalt

Describe physical changes associated with a malnourished state.

19. The nurse found the following assessment characteristics in the patient in the scenario and noted which ones that indicate a malnourished state? *(Select all that apply.)* *(746)*
    1. Weight loss
    2. Muscle atrophy
    3. Elevated temperature
    4. Dry hair that easily falls out
    5. Fat depletion in the waist, arms, and legs

20. What laboratory studies can be used to assess lean body mass? *(Select all that apply.)* *(746)*
    1. Ferritin
    2. Albumin
    3. Transferrin
    4. Prealbumin
    5. Retinol-binding protein

21. When providing patient teaching about kwashiorkor, which statements does the nurse include? *(Select all that apply.)* *(746)*
    1. "Kwashiorkor occurs because of a fat deficiency in the diet."
    2. "Patients with this condition receive adequate fats in the diet."
    3. "Patients with this condition receive adequate protein in the diet."
    4. "Patients with this condition receive adequate carbohydrates in the diet."
    5. "Patients with this condition are often difficult to recognize because they appear to be well-nourished."

Discuss nursing assessments and interventions required during the administration of enteral nutrition.

22. What are the general routines nurses use to monitor tube feedings? *(Select all that apply.)* *(748)*
    1. Checking tube placement
    2. Changing the tube feeding bag every 4 hours
    3. Monitoring for diarrhea or cramping
    4. Checking residual volumes of enteral feedings
    5. Performing daily weights and monitoring for signs of dehydration or overhydration

23. What assessments does the nurse perform prior to administering enteral nutrition? *(Select all that apply.)* *(750)*
    1. Assess daily weights.
    2. Assess bowel function.
    3. Assess for lactose intolerance.
    4. Assess the patency of the IV.
    5. Check laboratory results of Hgb, ALT, AST, and albumin.

24. How does the nurse administer a tube feeding that is prescribed to be given intermittently? *(750)*
    1. Administer 200 mL over 30 minutes using gravity.
    2. Slowly administer over 12-24 hours using a pump.
    3. Administer 200 mL over 5 minutes using a syringe.
    4. Administer 200 mL over 10 minutes using a pump.

Describe the advantages and disadvantages of nutrition by peripheral parenteral nutrition (PPN) and central parenteral nutrition (CPN).

25. What is the difference between PPN solutions and CPN solutions? *(Select all that apply.)* *(753)*
    1. CPN is used for patients who need nutritional support for 3-4 weeks; PPN is used for patients who require long-term nutritional support.
    2. PPN solutions consist of 5%-10% dextrose; CPN consists of 15%-25% glucose.
    3. CPN solutions must be administered through a central venous access line; PPN solutions may be administered through a peripheral line.
    4. CPN solutions contain electrolytes, vitamins, and minerals; PPN solutions contain electrolytes and vitamins.
    5. PPN solutions consist of 2%-5% amino acids; CPN solutions consist of 3.5%-15% amino acids.

26. Which adverse effects of parenteral feedings should be reported to the healthcare provider? *(Select all that apply.)* *(753-754)*
    1. Respiratory difficulty
    2. Rash, chills, and fever
    3. Hypoglycemia and/or hyperglycemia
    4. Infusion pump alarm for air in line
    5. 50 mL of solution remains in the bag after 24 hours

27. The nurse was discussing the advantages of enteral nutrition over parenteral nutrition with a patient who was going home with a gastrostomy port. Additional instruction was required after the patient made which statement? *(750)*
    1. "I know that this feeding will help stimulate my GI tract."
    2. "I will be getting all my nutrition through these feedings."
    3. "As I understand it, there is less of a chance of infection with this tube."
    4. "I understand these feedings are more expensive than if I had an IV drip for nutrition."

Herbal and Dietary Supplement Therapy

Answer Key: Textbook page references are provided as a guide for answering these questions. A complete answer key is provided to your instructor.

MATCHING

Match the supplement on the right with its use on the left.

Use

1. _____ a common beverage used to improve cognitive performance and stimulate the CNS

2. _____ research supports that it reduces cholesterol and triglyceride levels

3. _____ used as a digestive aid for bloating, and as an antispasmodic and antiinflammatory of the GI tract

4. _____ used to alleviate nausea and vomiting from a variety of causes

5. _____ used primarily as adjunctive therapy for chronic heart failure

6. _____ used to increase the body's resistance to stress

7. _____ frequently used as a coingredient in skin care products for healing sunburn

8. _____ used for restlessness and may promote sleep

9. _____ used to reduce the frequency and severity of migraine headaches

10. _____ used to treat short-term memory loss, headaches, dizziness, tinnitus, and emotional instability

11. _____ used orally to treat mild depression and to heal wounds

12. _____ used as a bronchodilator for asthma, a nasal decongestant, and a CNS stimulant

Supplement

a. aloe
b. chamomile
c. ephedra
d. feverfew
e. garlic
f. ginger
g. ginkgo
h. ginseng
i. green tea
j. St. John's wort
k. valerian
l. CoQ10

REVIEW QUESTIONS

Scenario: A 52-year-old woman came to the clinic complaining of joint pain, especially in her knees. She was told she may be getting degenerative joint disease. She told the nurse that she has been taking ginger and black cohosh.

Summarize the primary actions and potential uses of the herbal and dietary supplement products cited.

13. When a diabetic patient is taking aloe, it is most important for the nurse to assess the patient for the development of which condition? *(759)*
    1. Infection
    2. Hyperglycemia
    3. Hypokalemia
    4. Hypoglycemia

14. The nurse tells the patient in the scenario when the use of black cohosh would be contraindicated by making which statement? *(759)*
    1. "Black cohosh should not be used by patients who have arthritis conditions."
    2. "Black cohosh should not be used in the first two trimesters of pregnancy."
    3. "Black cohosh should not be used by patients who are immunocompromised."
    4. "Black cohosh should not be used by patients who are allergic to ragweed or asters."

15. What are common uses for chamomile? *(Select all that apply.)* **(760)**
    1. Alleviate nausea and vomiting
    2. Digestive agent for bloating
    3. An antiinflammatory for skin irritation
    4. An antispasmodic for menstrual cramps
    5. A mouthwash for minor mouth irritation or gum infections

16. A patient with which condition is most likely to benefit from the administration of echinacea? **(760)**
    1. Multiple sclerosis
    2. Systemic lupus erythematosus
    3. Viral respiratory tract infection
    4. Acquired immunodeficiency syndrome (AIDS)

17. What are common uses for feverfew? *(Select all that apply.)* **(761)**
    1. Alleviate nausea and vomiting
    2. Treatment of rheumatoid arthritis
    3. Reduce allergic response to ragweed
    4. Reduce the frequency and severity of migraine headaches
    5. Improve digestion and gastroesophageal reflux disease (GERD) symptoms

18. What common use for garlic is supported by scientific literature? **(762)**
    1. Alleviate nausea and vomiting
    2. Reduce fever and inflammation
    3. Reduce cholesterol and triglycerides
    4. Improve digestion and GERD symptoms

19. The patient in the scenario was asking the nurse what effects ginger has as an herbal preparation. Which statement would be an appropriate response from the nurse? *(Select all that apply.)* **(762-763)**
    1. "Ginger works as an aphrodisiac."
    2. "Ginger has no medicinal effects, so it basically works like a placebo."
    3. "Ginger has been used for centuries to alleviate nausea and vomiting."
    4. "Ginger has some modest effects in reducing the inflammation associated with rheumatoid arthritis."
    5. "Ginger has been known to reduce allergic reactions in patients with hayfever."

20. What is *Ginkgo biloba* extract commonly used for? *(Select all that apply.)* **(763)**
    1. To increase cerebral blood flow, particularly in geriatric patients
    2. To improve erectile dysfunction secondary to antidepressant therapy
    3. To improve walking distance in patients with intermittent claudication
    4. To improve hearing in patients with hearing impairment due to poor circulation to the ears
    5. To improve eyesight in patients with vision impairment due to poor circulation to the eyes

21. Which herb is also known by other names that include *red berry, tartar root, five fingers,* and *aralia quinquefolia?* **(763)**
    1. Goldenseal
    2. Ginseng
    3. Valerian
    4. Feverfew

22. Which herb has its active ingredients contained in plant alkaloids, the most active of which are hydrastine and berberine? **(764)**
    1. St. John's wort
    2. Ginseng
    3. Goldenseal
    4. Green tea

23. Of the ingredients that are active in green tea, which causes adverse effects such as anxiety, nervousness, and insomnia? **(765)**
    1. Caffeine
    2. Gallic acid
    3. Catechins
    4. Ascorbic acid

24. Which herb is used for treatment of mild depression? **(765)**
    1. Valerian
    2. Green tea
    3. St. John's wort
    4. Ginseng

25. Which statements does the nurse include when teaching a patient about St. John's wort? *(Select all that apply.)* **(765)**
    1. "The active ingredients of St. John's wort are unknown."
    2. "St. John's wort is a safe drug for anyone with depression."
    3. "There are no adverse effects associated with the use of St. John's wort."
    4. "St. John's wort may cause photosensitivity, so individuals using it should avoid overexposure to the sun."
    5. "Patients who take other serotonin stimulants should not take St. John's wort without consulting their healthcare provider."

26. Which are common uses for valerian? *(Select all that apply.)* **(766)**
    1. Laxative
    2. Sleep aid
    3. Digestive aid
    4. Alleviate restlessness
    5. Reduce inflammation

27. The provitamin coenzyme Q10 can be found in every living cell and accumulates in high levels in organs that have high energy requirements such as what? *(Select all that apply.)* **(766)**
    1. Lung
    2. Brain
    3. Liver
    4. Heart
    5. Pancreas

28. Which herbal preparation is thought to enhance muscle performance for short bouts of intense exercise? *(767)*
    1. Creatine
    2. Melatonin
    3. Coenzyme Q10
    4. Gamma-hydroxybutyrate

29. Why is gamma-hydroxybutyrate (GHB) available as a prescription-only product used for narcolepsy? *(768)*
    1. The adverse effects are hypertension and tachycardia.
    2. The effects of its blood-thinning properties make it too dangerous.
    3. It easily produces symptoms of nausea, vomiting, and diarrhea.
    4. It has been used as a date rape drug added to alcoholic drinks.

30. Which herbal compound is found in tomatoes, watermelon, and pink grapefruit? *(768)*
    1. Lycopene
    2. Melatonin
    3. Ginseng
    4. Chamomile

31. Which preparation is naturally produced from serotonin and secreted by the pineal gland? *(768)*
    1. Lycopene
    2. Melatonin
    3. Policosanol
    4. Omega-3 fatty acids

32. Which action is policosanol used to produce? *(769)*
    1. Decrease pulse rate
    2. Lower blood sugar
    3. Lower cholesterol levels
    4. Lower blood pressure

33. Which are sources of omega-3 fatty acids? *(Select all that apply.)* *(769)*
    1. Tuna
    2. Sardines
    3. Soybeans
    4. Flaxseed
    5. Peanuts

34. Which conditions are possible indications for the use of S-adenosylmethionine (SAM-e)? *(Select all that apply.)* *(770)*
    1. Infection
    2. Depression
    3. Osteoarthritis
    4. Diabetes mellitus
    5. Fibromyalgia

Describe the interactions between commonly used herbal and dietary supplement products and prescription medications.

35. The patient in the scenario is on hormone replacement therapy to treat symptoms associated with menopause and to prevent osteoporosis. She also takes medication to control high blood pressure. She asks the nurse about the risks of taking black cohosh. What is the best response by the nurse? *(760)*
    1. "Black cohosh works by stimulating the body to produce its own natural testosterone."
    2. "Studies have found that black cohosh is an excellent herb for women to treat symptoms of menopause that are not controlled by hormone replacement therapy."
    3. "High blood pressure will be lowered with the use of black cohosh, so you won't need to take your high blood pressure pills any longer."
    4. "Black cohosh may cause added antihypertensive effects when taken with medication to lower blood pressure. Consult your healthcare provider before adding black cohosh to your treatment regimen."

36. Which herbal supplement affects platelet aggregation and therefore should be used with caution for patients taking antiplatelet medications? *(762)*
    1. Garlic
    2. Ephedra
    3. Melatonin
    4. Black cohosh

37. The nurse needs to caution patients who drink alcohol or take benzodiazepines and sleep aids that the adverse effect of CNS depression may occur with the addition of which herbal product? *(769)*
    1. creatine
    2. melatonin
    3. policosanol
    4. omega-3 fatty acids

Substance Abuse

Answer Key: Textbook page references are provided as a guide for answering these questions. A complete answer key is provided to your instructor.

MATCHING
Match the slang drug name on the right with the substances of abuse on the left.

Substance of Abuse

1. _____ heroin
2. _____ nicotine
3. _____ cocaine
4. _____ marijuana
5. _____ LSD
6. _____ PCP
7. _____ alcohol

Slang Name

a. acid
b. blast
c. booze
d. weed
e. angel dust
f. China white
g. chew

REVIEW QUESTIONS

Scenario: A 26-year-old woman came into the clinic for a prenatal exam and was obviously intoxicated.

Identify the differences between mild, moderate, and severe substance abuse disorder.

8. The term *social impairment* is described as having which components? *(Select all that apply.)* **(774)**
   1. Craving exhibited by a powerful urge for the substance
   2. Development of withdrawal symptoms when blood levels decline
   3. Continuation of substance use in spite of persistent social problems
   4. Reduction or cessation of important social, occupational, or recreational pursuits because of substance use
   5. Failure to meet responsibilities at work, school, or home because of recurrent substance use

9. When four or five symptoms of substance use disorders are present, the patient is classified as having what? **(773)**
   1. A mild substance abuse disorder
   2. A moderate substance abuse disorder
   3. A severe substance abuse disorder
   4. A true addictive substance disorder

10. What symptoms are included in the description of a severe substance abuse disorder? *(Select all that apply.)* **(773)**
    1. The use of illicit substances
    2. An overwhelming compulsion to use the substance
    3. Feeling depressed when not using the substance
    4. A tolerance for higher amounts of the substance
    5. Withdrawal symptoms on discontinuation of the substance

Differentiate between the screening instruments for substance use disorders.

11. What questionnaire will the nurse use as a quick screening instrument for assessment of alcohol abuse for the patient in the scenario? **(775)**
    1. MMPI
    2. API
    3. CAGE
    4. DUSI

12. What is one disadvantage of many of the screening instruments used for assessment of substance abuse? **(775)**
    1. They cannot differentiate between alcohol problems or drug problems.
    2. They have been designed as self-assessment tools and require the use of a computer.

3. They were developed using adult male patients and have not been validated in other populations.
4. They have many lengthy questions and are not specific enough to detect the difference between excessive drinking and alcoholism.

13. Screening instruments used by healthcare professionals for patients who are suspected of substance abuse are divided into which four categories? (*Select all that apply.*) **(775)**
    1. Alcohol abuse screening
    2. Brief drug abuse screening
    3. Lengthy drug abuse screening
    4. Comprehensive drug abuse screening
    5. Drug and alcohol abuse screening for use with adolescents

Cite the responsibilities of professionals who suspect substance abuse by a colleague.

14. What is the prevalence of substance abuse by healthcare professionals? **(775)**
    1. Unheard of in this profession
    2. Similar to the general population
    3. Much lower than the general population
    4. Much higher than the general population

15. What should a healthcare professional do if he or she suspects a colleague of being impaired on the job? **(775)**
    1. Do nothing, but keep an eye on the colleague.
    2. Confront the individual about the suspicion.
    3. Make a confidential report to the supervisor.
    4. Inform all coworkers about the situation.

16. A nurse was discussing her suspicions about a coworker to her supervisor and asked if the coworker was going to lose her job. What is an appropriate response by the supervisor? **(778)**
    1. "No, we cannot afford to fire anyone at this time; we are too understaffed."
    2. "Yes, but she could always reapply for the job after she has been out for a year."
    3. "No, not at this point. The next step is to have this person enter a treatment program."
    4. "Yes, unfortunately that is the way it works. We cannot have someone impaired on the job."

Explain the primary long-term goals in the treatment of substance abuse.

17. When providing teaching to the patient in the scenario about the effects of substance use and abuse with pregnancy, which statements does the nurse include? (*Select all that apply.*) **(788)**
    1. "Using alcohol and drugs while pregnant has a strong likelihood of harming the baby before and after birth."
    2. "Infants of drug addicts must be monitored closely for symptoms of withdrawal after delivery."

3. "Using alcohol and drugs during pregnancy has a high likelihood of causing the need for induction of labor due to the fetus being postterm."
4. "Alcohol and drug use during pregnancy has been associated with potentially fatal bleeding disorders."
5. "Babies of mothers who used alcohol during pregnancy have a higher incidence of behavioral problems later in life."

18. What are the long-term goals in treating substance abuse? (*Select all that apply.*) **(780)**
    1. Maintenance of social functioning
    2. Reduction in the severity of relapse
    3. Reduction in the frequency of relapse
    4. Abstinence in the use of the substance being abused
    5. Reduction in the use of the substance being abused

19. When patients are participating in organizations such as Alcoholics Anonymous or Narcotics Anonymous, what types of resources are available to them? (*Select all that apply.*) **(781)**
    1. Networking
    2. Role modeling
    3. Advice on abstinence
    4. Money for expenses
    5. 24-hour help available when a craving occurs

Identify the withdrawal symptoms for major substances that are commonly abused.

20. Which are signs and symptoms of opioid intoxication? (*Select all that apply.*) **(783-784)**
    1. Apathy
    2. Inappropriate behaviors
    3. Impaired judgment
    4. Miosis, slurred speech
    5. Avoidance of dangerous situations

21. What drug class is used to treat alcohol withdrawal symptoms? **(782)**
    1. Adrenergic agents
    2. Benzodiazepines
    3. Cholinergic agents
    4. Anticholinergic agents

22. When working with a patient who is withdrawing from long-term use of amphetamines, the nurse expects the patient to exhibit which signs/symptoms? (*Select all that apply.*) **(785)**
    1. Insomnia
    2. Fatigue
    3. Severe depression
    4. Loss of memory
    5. Inability to manipulate information